THE COLORS of OKLAHOMA MUSIC

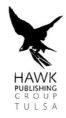

HAWK
PUBLISHING
GROUP
TULSA

FROM THE BLUE DEVILS
★ TO RED DIRT ★

THE COLORS of OKLAHOMA MUSIC

BY JOHN WOOLEY

LIBRARY OF CONGRESS CATALOGING-IN-PUBLICATION DATA

Wooley, John
From Blue Devils to Red Dirt: The Colors of Oklahoma Music / John Wooley
ISBN 1-930709-61-7
LOC #2006928192
Copyright 2006 by John Wooley

All rights reserved under International and Pan-American Copyright Conventions. No part of this book may be reproduced, stored in a retrieval system or transmitted in any form by an electronic, mechanical, photocopying, recording means or otherwise, without prior written permission of the author.

Published in the United States by HAWK Publishing Group.
HAWK Publishing Group
7107 South Yale Avenue #345
Tulsa, OK 74136
918-492-3677
hawkpub.com
HAWK and colophon are trademarks belonging to the HAWK Publishing Group.

Interior and Cover Design by
Müllerhaus Publishing Arts, Inc. | MullerhausPubArts.com

Printed in the United States of America.
9 8 7 6 5 4 3 2 1

The purpose of the Oklahoma Arts Institute (OAI) is to provide programs of excellence in arts education for Oklahoma and the region in order to develop future artists and art audiences while enhancing the quality of life for all Oklahomans. In 1991, the Oklahoma legislature passed a joint resolution designating the Institute "Oklahoma's Official School of the Arts."

Since 1976, the OAI has recruited nationally-renowned artists to teach fine arts programs for talented Oklahoma youth and continuing education workshops for adults. Oklahoma high school students are selected through a statewide competitive audition process for a two-week, intensive summer arts academy. Each fall, educators, professional artists, and students gather for four-day weekend workshops in the literary, visual, and performing arts.

The Oklahoma Arts Institute is part of a unique public/private partnership. Major funding is provided by private donors secured by the Oklahoma Arts Institute, with matching funds from the Oklahoma State Department of Education and additional support from the Oklahoma Arts Council and the Oklahoma Department of Tourism and Recreation. The generosity of Institute donors provides scholarships for the high school students and teachers.

In 1906, ONEOK's founders began providing safe, reliable energy to Oklahomans. Today, they continue the tradition of excellence and community involvement, celebrating 100 years of service to our great state.

This book, published in the fall of 2006, was made possible by a joint endeavor of ONEOK, the Oklahoma Centennial Commission, and the Institute in order to commemorate Oklahoma's one hundredth birthday and proudly lead the way into the next century.

These worthwhile projects are the cornerstones of a renewed commitment to support Oklahoma literature and authors. All profits generated from the books will be used to publish additional projects that bring to life the heart and soul of Oklahoma.

DEDICATION

In 1983, I was hired to write about music for the *Tulsa World*. Twenty-three years later, I'm still writing about it. Working for the *World* has allowed me to encounter scores of musicians connected to our state, and to explore their motives and creative visions, their interconnectedness, their lasting contributions. If not for the couple of decades of crafting music-related stories for the newspaper, I would've been supremely under-qualified to take on an assignment like this one. And if the *World* hadn't been gracious enough to permit me to draw freely from the thousands of stories I've contributed to the paper over the years, I would've never been able to meet this book's deadline.

For those reasons, and others, I respectfully dedicate this work to the *Tulsa World* itself, which has brought me into the orbits of hundreds of performers of all kinds, allowing me to make a living by bringing a little back to share from each and every one. When it comes to Oklahoma music, I don't for a minute think I have all the answers. Thanks to the *World*, though, I've been able to collect a lot of pieces of the puzzle.

What follows is my attempt to put them together.

ACKNOWLEDGEMENTS

Except where noted, all quotes used in this text come from interviews I've conducted, mostly for the *Tulsa World*, beginning in the early '80s. In addition to giving thanks to all of the artists and others I've interviewed, I want to single out *World Scene* editor Cathy Logan, my HAWK(eyed) editor Jodie Nida, HAWK Publishing Group head Bill Bernhardt, Doug Miller and all the talented graphic designers at Müllerhaus Publishing Arts, CEO Chuck Cissel and executive assistant Bettie Downing at the Oklahoma Jazz Hall of Fame, jazz musician and historian John Hamill, writer and editor Thomas Conner, Leon Russell biographer Steve Todoroff, and George Lang, assistant entertainment editor at the *Daily Oklahoman*. All of these people helped fill in some blanks in the manuscript, amplified what I already had, or made substantial contributions in other ways, and I'm grateful.

I'm also deeply indebted to the Oklahoma Centennial Committee, whose members green-lighted this project. I hope it fulfills the trust they placed in me. As I wrote, I was always aware I was writing for posterity, which made me want to be doubly sure I was getting it right.

Finally, I should note that beyond the books and other resources cited individually within these pages, I found the website *www.allmusic.com* very helpful for checking both biographical information and chart positions of records.

INTRODUCTION

In its first hundred years, Oklahoma has gifted the world with a rich and colorful array of music stars, from the hardscrabble, spirited band that foreshadowed Count Basie's Orchestra to the No. 1 pop music act of the '90s. Those would be the Oklahoma City Blue Devils and Garth Brooks, respectively, separated by six decades but united in their Sooner State origins. And just about here is the point where the author should begin a spiel about the great diversity of our musicians over the decades, about how we've produced notable artists in virtually every musical genre, etc. etc.

Indeed, all of that's true. But for this author, who's been studying and writing about Oklahoma's music in many of its permutations for more than a quarter of a century, there's a nagging question dogging this journey of musical discovery. Sure, it tells us, Oklahoma's produced scores of great performers. But so have our neighbors in the big state to our immediate south. (If you don't believe it, just ask them.) And California. And Iowa, Montana, and Maine. When you think about it, you'd be hard pressed to find an American state that can't lay claim to at least a few musical greats. Then what, exactly, makes our state so different?

That's the big question. And when you consider it, the whole notion of a book about Oklahoma music changes focus. Instead of simply being about the musical Okies whose talent and ambition propelled them to the top of their respective fields, it has to become something more. It has to take a shot, at least, at answering that question, as well as the related ones that spring up in its wake: Are we really all that different? And if we are, then how are we different?

As the author of this book, and an Oklahoma resident for virtually all my life, I've become convinced that there's a strong case to be made for our musical uniqueness. I believe that we are, indeed, different, and that the difference has a lot to do not only with the interweaving of musical genres unique to our part of the country, but also the character of the state and its people—a character burnished in the crucible of the Dust Bowl of the 1930s and carried in the cultural memory of Oklahomans to this day.

There aren't a lot of people left who remember that awful time, when there was as much land swirling in the sky as there was underfoot, and desperate families hit the highways or stayed and starved. Yet, out of those terrible years came the kinds of stories my mother still tells, about how her own father, who worked on an oil lease and thus was blessed with a steady income, would go into town every payday and buy two sacks each of staples like sugar and flour, sharing equally with the farm family down the road, who had nothing and no prospects. Put in simple terms, there was an innate obligation to take care of your neighbor, not to grind your heel in his face on your way up the ladder of success.

Because my grandfather shared with those outside his family, there was no disposable income for his kids, who had to learn to make do with what they had. But while he made sure to take care of the basic needs of his immediate family, he also realized—as the Joads ultimately did in John Steinbeck's testament to the Oklahoma spirit, the classic Dust Bowl novel *The Grapes of Wrath*—that "family" in no way meant only your blood relatives. His children understood, and when they grew up, they passed it on.

It's a sublimely Christian notion in a religious land, most famously and directly expressed in the songs of Okemah's Woody Guthrie—and, in a different but no less powerful way, by the Tulsa-based Bob Wills and His Texas Playboys. Both of those iconic Oklahoma-music figures tackled the Dust Bowl and the surrounding Great Depression in real time, applying two different philosophies—which we'll deal with later in these pages—to uplift the poor and dispirited, again and again.

Even before those dark days, however, the notion of community permeated our state's pioneering jazz band, the Oklahoma City Blue Devils.

In his book *One O'Clock Jump: The Unforgettable History of the Oklahoma City Blue Devils* (Beacon Press, 2006), author Douglas Henry Daniels notes that the members of the Blue Devils, from their early '20s beginnings, were guys who emphasized taking care of one another. "The 'all for one and one for all' attitude of the bandsmen," writes Daniels, "mirrored the community spirit of the Oklahoma frontier."

Flash forward seventy years to the 2005 installment of the Red Dirt Rangers' annual Christmas concert at Tulsa's Cain's Ballroom—the former home of Bob Wills—where the wildly cheering packed house is getting a full-throttle seminar in the Stillwater-forged, deeply Oklahoman music known as Red Dirt. On this particular night, the headline act is Cross Canadian Ragweed, a captivating rock-edged band that roared out of Stillwater to national fame. As the show goes on, other Red Dirt performers wander on and off the stage, performing with CCR in a spirit of kinship, of family, a feeling made all the more poignant when one finds out that the group—which commands somewhere in the middle five figures per show—waived any guaranteed fee for this job, instead sharing the take at the door with the other Red Dirt performers on the bill. And when, at the end of the evening, this hard-rocking outfit plays a Bob Wills song with both joy and respect, the circle, on this night, seems wonderfully complete.

That's the kind of thing this book is about. It's not intended to be a complete, or even a near-complete, listing of the musical giants our state has produced. (For that, check out the *Oklahoma Music Guide* by George O. Carney and Hugh W. Foley Jr, published by New Forums Press in 2003 and still available at this writing.) You'll find many of those figures in these pages, of course, as we look at the forces they captured here at home, mixed together, and released like clouds of newly colored butterflies through the years, delighting us as well as countless folks beyond our borders.

But what I hope you also get from this book is something deeper—a feeling for, and understanding of, the music that courses through our land like blood and sparking nerves, representing us and our changing faces, thoughts, and feelings while remaining true to the good and natural impulses of community and sharing that helped get our forebears through the Dust Bowl some three generations ago. From the Blue Devils to Red Dirt, Oklahoma's music has unfolded in some fascinating ways.

Let's look at them together.

—**John Wooley**

1
CHAPTER ONE
THE OKLAHOMA CITY BLUE DEVILS — AND BEYOND

ON Sundays, my church, CME Church, [was] just one block from *the* street . . . Northeast Second Street, about three hundred block. They called that Deep Deuce and that was the main spot for the black community . . .

They had kind of a little headquarters there where the cats would gang up and get ready to go to the gig and play. Everybody would just meet there and they get in their cars and go hit it . . .

. . . Count Basie and the Blue Devils and all that stuff like that, they all knew each other and everything [was] family-like . . .

   —trumpeter and pianist **Buddy Anderson**,
     quoted in *Goin' to Kansas City* by Nathan W. Pearson Jr.
     (University of Illinois Press, 1987)

THERE was such a team spirit among those guys [The Oklahoma City Blue Devils], and it came out in their music.

   —William "Count" Basie, in *Good Morning Blues:*
     The Autobiography of Count Basie, as told to
     Albert Murray (Random House, 1985)

In 1923, a traveling show featuring a popular vaudevillian named Billy King stopped at Oklahoma City's Aldridge Theatre, a venue on Second Street, squarely in the area of the city known as Deep Deuce. Deep Deuce was the nickname of the business and residential area where much of Oklahoma City's African-American population lived and worked at the time. It was also the area that gave birth to one of the most influential early jazz bands in the country, the Oklahoma City Blue Devils. While the group only recorded two songs in its decade-long career, it provided the model and some of the personnel for bands that would come to define the Kansas City jazz sound, including the orchestras of Bennie Moten and Count Basie.

In his book-length study *One O'Clock Jump: The Unforgettable History of the Oklahoma City Blue Devils* (cited in our introduction), author Douglas Henry Daniels notes that a band called the Blue Devils Orchestra accompanied King for the duration of his Aldridge Theatre gig, and that the group that contained many of the musicians who'd later be cited as the founders of the Oklahoma City Blue Devils. It's unclear, however, how many of these players blew into town with King as a part of the roadshow, and how many came out of the Deep Deuce scene, an area already rich with good music and outstanding musicians.

Daniels writes that this Blue Devils Orchestra "was perhaps a temporary affair," which means that it could've been a collection of area musicians assembled for this particular stop, or a few regional stops, on King's roadshow tour. (The practice of hiring area musicians to back local shows by a touring performer—either as players supplementing a core road band or comprising a complete backing group—has been a common practice for many decades, continuing to this day.)

Daniels also speculates on the origins of the Blue Devils' name, feeling that it was a way of tipping African-American audiences to the fact that the band members were also black. (He cites former Blue Devil Eddie Durham as backup for that theory). But he also takes the band's frontier origins into consideration. "Blue devils," Daniels writes, "are the sharp barbs on barbed wire, [so] the band's name carried the implication that they looked and played sharp enough to cut." Then there's the idea, advanced by the great Oklahoma City writer Ralph Ellison (of *Invisible Man* fame), that "blue devils" was a name given to the scofflaws who cut down barbed wire during the range wars of the late 1800s, something the band members might well have known and appropriated in order to convey a certain outlaw image. Finally, there's the whole connotation of "blues" in the band's name, Blues music, after all, was quite familiar to

Southwestern black audiences at the time.

Although author Daniels offers some intriguing speculations, we don't really know with certainty why and how the band got its name. What we do know is that in its ten years of existence, it was home at one time or another to such influential jazzmen as the trumpeter Oran "Hot Lips" Page, vocalist Jimmy Rushing, saxophonists Lester "Pres" Young and Don Byas, and famed pianist and bandleader Count Basie, who's said to have built his sound and his group right along the lines of the Oklahoma City Blue Devils. It was a band that played for both black and white audiences—not together, of course, except under special circumstances—and wowed them both. And it was an aggregation whose reputation among other musicians far exceeded its national fame. Renowned jazz drummer Jo Jones was undoubtedly speaking for many of his musical comrades when he was quoted by author and noted jazz critic Stanley Dance in *The World of Count Basie*, (Random House, 1985). "The greatest band I ever heard," Jones stated, "was Mr. Walter Page's Blue Devils."

Page, a Missourian who could play tuba, bass, and baritone sax with equal facility, was one of the originators of the group, a member of the Blue Devils Orchestra who played the 1923 King show in Oklahoma City and stayed at the helm of the band as it metamorphosed into the Oklahoma City Blue Devils. Like many of his comrades, the college-educated Page (apparently not related to later bandmate Hot Lips Page, a Texas native) eventually left the Blue Devils for the Kansas City scene and Bennie Moten, with whom he had played before becoming a Blue Devil. However, Page was a linchpin of the band throughout its glory years, leading them through endless dancehall nights, long stretches of road, and lots of bandstand battles with other groups.

The latter pursuit, in which two or more bands competed for the approval of their audiences, seemed to have been something the members of the Blue Devils particularly enjoyed. Hanging in the Oklahoma Jazz Hall of Fame in downtown Tulsa is a big photo-illustrated advertisement from the November 23, 1928 edition of the *Kansas City Call* that indicates the entertainment value inherent in this sort of show. It trumpets "Walter

"BLUE DEVILS," DANIELS WRITES, "ARE THE SHARP BARBS ON BARBED WIRE, [SO] THE BAND'S NAME CARRIED THE IMPLICATION THAT THEY LOOKED AND PLAYED SHARP ENOUGH TO CUT."

Page & His Famous Blue Devils vs. George Lee and His Novelty Singing Orchestra," asking in big type, "Can George E. Lee outplay the 'Blue Devils'? Can he outsing James Rushing?"

Like Lee's outfit in Kansas City and the Dallas-based Alphonso Trent Orchestra, to name a couple of the better-known examples, The Oklahoma City Blue Devils were a "territory band." That meant that, with a few exceptions, they never strayed more than a state or two away from their home base. For years, the Blue Devils spent their winters playing at Oklahoma City's

year on Vocalion, a well-known label.

The Oklahoma City Blue Devils were a commonwealth band. That means that while Walter Page and others managed as well as played in the group and sometimes appended their name to it (they occasionally were billed as "Walter Page and His Famous Blue Devils") every man received an equal amount of money and had a say in decisions affecting the band. Musicians know that a commonwealth situation demands a certain amount of altruism and often works better in theory than in fact, with many a promising com-

"OKLAHOMA MUSICIANS ARE DIFFERENT NOT ONLY FOR THE INFLUENCES THEY'VE TAKEN AND SHAPED AND BLENDED INTO NEW KINDS OF SOUNDS, BUT ALSO FOR THE ATTITUDE THEY'VE BROUGHT TO THEIR WORK AND THEIR LIVES WHILE THEY'RE DOING IT."

Ritz Ballroom and other in-state venues, venturing to dancehall jobs at other times of the year on a circuit that included Nebraska, Texas, Missouri and Arkansas. Of course, Kansas City was a frequent stop. In fact, it was during a Kansas City engagement in 1929 that the Oklahoma City Blue Devils cut their only record. One side was "Squabblin'," a mid-tempo instrumental. The other featured Jimmy Rushing singing a tune called "Blue Devil Blues." The disc came out that

monwealth group brought down by infighting and side-choosing, or even by the recalcitrance of a single member. Although Blue Devils came and went, as is the case with any band that lasts a substantial number of years, the group was apparently successful at resolving problems and challenges within the commonwealth structure. This undoubtedly had a lot to do with their "all for one and one for all" philosophy—author Daniels maintains that the men appropriated the famous motto from the silent-movie version of *The Three Musketeers*—in which taking care of one another was of paramount importance.

Like the Oklahoma folks who learned about brotherhood and selflessness when the Dust Bowl mercilessly compounded the soul-grinding effects of the Great Depression—which hit, incidentally, about midway through the Blue Devils' life—the band members forged strong bonds, in part by simply surviving together the challenges faced by African-American road musicians crisscrossing the middle of the country in order to make a living.

In *One O'Clock Jump*, Daniels cites a 1965 *Downbeat* magazine story profiling Oklahoma City native and one-time Blue Devil Jimmy Rushing. "We weren't making money, but we were all friends," Rushing told interviewer Ruth McNamara, recalling his days with the outfit. "If one of the boys needed money—like his wife needed coal or had to pay the gas bill—we'd take the amount necessary out of the gross, give it to him, and send him home and split down the leavings among the rest of us."

Rushing's statement beautifully illustrates the central thesis of this book—that Oklahoma musicians are different not only for the influences they've taken and shaped and blended into new kinds of sounds, but also for the attitude they've brought to their work and their lives while they're doing it. It was and is something that transcends simple decency, although that's a part of it.

It goes far deeper, though, into the deep-seated spirituality of the state's people—most of whom, as was the case with the Blue Devils and their friends—know what the *New Testament* has to say about extending mercy, compassion, and aid to those who need it.

While the spiritual part of the Blue Devils' legacy made itself felt in the jazz scene that followed their dissolution, most notably in Count Basie's supremely successful swing orchestra, the musical part of their heritage was just as important—especially as an influence on the Kansas City jazz style. In her book *The Jazz of the Southwest* (University of Texas Press, 1998), author Jean A. Boyd notes that the Blue Devils band "was famous for its competitive spirit—band members preferred battle dances and jam sessions to any other performing context—and its loose, free-swinging rhythmic approach." Both of those things, she believes, eventually changed the sound of Kansas City jazz, which at the time was exemplified by Bennie Moten and his orchestra.

"When Kansas City bandleader Bennie Moten could not beat the Blue Devils in jam sessions," Boyd writes, "he hired them all, and in the process transformed his band's rather stilted rhythmic approach into a more energized swing."

It was, she adds, a different sound than the jazz bands from the northeast part of the country, thanks to the influence of the Blue Devils and others from the Oklahoma-Texas area.

One reason that southwestern bands felt a four-beat swing rhythm, while bands in the Northeast struggled with a rigid and less liberated two-beat approach, may be traced to the loose-limbed, highly improvised blues tradition that was fundamental to south-western jazz. Swing jazz probably originated in the rhythm sections of southwestern bands, but because of their limited recording opportunities and only local recognition, they are afforded almost no credit for helping to invent the style.

In their definition of Kansas City's jazz, found in *Jazz: The Rough Guide* (Rough Guides Ltd, 1995), authors Ian Carr, Digby Fairweather, and Brian Priestley connect that sound directly to Kansas City:

Early eastern bands such as Fletcher Henderson, Duke Ellington and even McKinney's in Detroit attempted an extrovert but neatly organized version of jazz, justified in hindsight by the inclusion of solos, and so at first did Bennie Moten. But the "territory bands" on which he drew for his sidemen had a rougher and more primitive blues-based style that gave the ensemble work more spontaneity, and eventually even introduced head [unwritten] arrangements. The fact that these were little more than riffs, and that opening themes were often interchangeable with backings for soloists, actually gave Kansas City bands (especially Count Basie's) greater stylistic unity and freedom. It is no coincidence that rhythmically repetitive riff-making was so central, for, in rhythm-section work too, the relaxed cohesion of the New Orleans style found a new home in Kansas City.

Jo Jones, Basie's drummer during the orchestra's golden age of the '30s and early '40s, gave the Oklahoma City Blue Devils direct credit—or at least *half*-credit—for the Kansas City sound exemplified by his former boss. He's quoted in Albert Murray's *Stomping the Blues* as saying, "When Bennie Moten's two beat one and three rhythm and the two and four of Walter Page's Blue Devils came together in the Basie band, there was an even flow of one-two-three-four."

"The best way I can explain it," said jazz-piano legend Jay McShann in a conversation before his 1999 induction into the Oklahoma Jazz Hall of Fame, "is that the first jazz, the New Orleans jazz, was two-beat—dum, dum . . . dum, dum. Then, Basie came through with that thing, that Kansas City thing, which was four beats—dum, dum, dum, dum. And it worked much better with what the Southwestern musicians were putting down, because they always did the blues with that beat—and a little bit of gospel.

"It's like they say at this thing here," he added, motioning to indicate the Oklahoma Jazz Hall of

Fame. "It's jazz, blues, and gospel. Kansas City jazz is built on that—built on the blues."

For a visual and musical representation of what McShann was talking about, the reader is referred to the Bruce Ricker documentary *The Last of the Blue Devils* (1980), which combines vintage interviews with and music from such famed Blue Devils as Walter Page and Lester Young with newer footage of Basie, McShann, and others. It's available on DVD from Kino Video.

Although McShann's life and work came directly out of the Blue Devils tradition, he was too young to be a Blue Devil. He was, however, an Oklahoman, born and raised in a town that's remarkable for the number of jazz greats it has produced—not Oklahoma City, but one best-known instead for a late 1960s down-home anthem from one of country music's greatest talents.

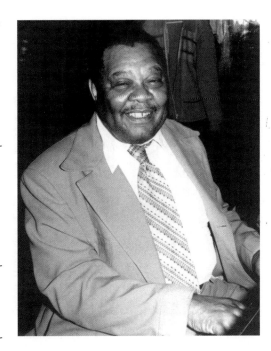

Jay McShann

> **Muskogee and Oklahoma City were sort of stopping-off points. A musician might have enough money to make it halfway, and then he'd get off the train at Oklahoma City, broke, and work around the area until he had enough money to go on. It was the same way with the route from New Orleans to Kansas City. People who made it halfway stopped off at Muskogee.**
>
> —*Dr. Guy Logsdon,* MUSIC HISTORIAN AND AUTHOR

The Oklahoma Music Hall of fame, established in 1996, is located not in Oklahoma City or Tulsa, the state's two largest cities, but in the smaller northeastern Oklahoma city of Muskogee, immortalized in the 1969 Merle Haggard mega-hit, "Okie From Muskogee" (written with his drummer Eddie Burris, after some of the band members glimpsed the town's name on a highway sign through their tour bus window). Fittingly, the hall of fame is headquartered in a former depot, on the old railroad lines ridden in the '20s and '30s by African-American jazz and blues musicians, many of whom stopped off in Muskogee for a few days—or longer. As the brilliant jazz guitarist and Muskogee native Barney Kessel remembered

Jay McShann

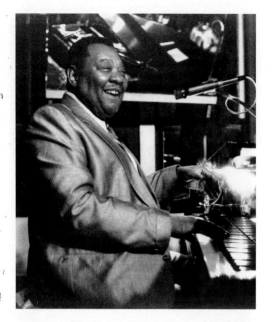

in a 1985 interview, "There were a great number of black musicians in Muskogee who had come in from Kansas City. They knew musicians like we know football players, and when they moved to Muskogee they brought that legacy with them. Everybody I played with in Muskogee had heard of [Oklahoma City jazz-guitar innovator] Charlie Christian before he ever joined Benny Goodman.

"These people had moved from Kansas City because they couldn't make a living," he added. "They were kind of second-string musicians, still very good, but not good enough to make it in that tremendously competitive jazz scene in Kansas City. That place was rich with club after club after club. It was as much a center for jazz music as ancient Athens was for philosophy—that's how important it was. So they had migrated simply to survive. They all had day jobs, but they would play dances three or four times a week."

What made Muskogee such a jazz town in the '20s and '30s? For one thing, it was, as Logsdon noted at the first of this section, a stop that lay almost halfway between two of the nation's jazz centers, New Orleans and Kansas City (although a lot more Muskogee players worked in the latter scene than the former). When the subject came up in interviews through the years, Jay McShann would invariably mention the town's excellent public-school music programs, as well as some of the Muskogee musicians who'd made it in Kansas City but still returned from time to time to play for the home folks.

One of these was Clarence Love, who led a Kansas City-based orchestra that emphasized the "sweet" (as opposed to "hot") style of swing music. "When we were in school, if they were gonna play a dance [in Muskogee], they'd come by and play a couple of pep songs at the school," recalled McShann in 1996, talking about Love's outfit. "Clarence Love always had good players, and I'd listen to these cats play, man. A lot of times, bands would play off the backs of trucks down there, to advertise stuff. The trumpets'd be blowin' and the whole thing, and I loved it. Music's a funny thing. You can hear it in the air, you know. You can hear

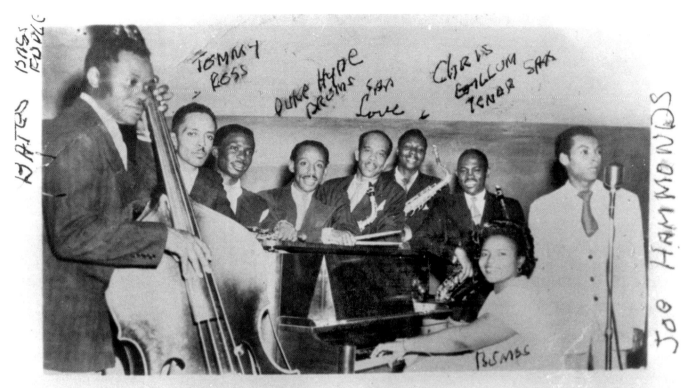

CLARENCE LOVE and his BIG TEN BALLROOM ORCHESTRA.

Clarence Love and his Big Ten Ballroom Orchestra

it before it gets to you."

There was lots of music in the air in the late '20s and the 1930s, while McShann and other nascent musicians were growing up in the town. But again the question arises: Why Muskogee?

Some historians feel that it has a lot to do with the removal of the Five Civilized Tribes to Indian Territory, which, in 1907, would merge with Oklahoma Territory—the area bounding it on the west—to become the state of Oklahoma. Many in the tribes were slaveholders, and when they were relocated to Indian Territory, they brought their slaves along. When slavery was abolished following the Civil War, many African-Americans freed by the people of the Five Civilized Tribes stayed in what became eastern Oklahoma—an area that includes Muskogee.

"Most of Oklahoma's jazzmen were black musicians, and many of these black jazzmen were freedmen," explained historian Logsdon. "They had their roots here before much white settlement came in. Also, there was talk of making Oklahoma an all-black state in the 1890s and

1900s, which attracted a lot of black people."

As a result of this African-American influx 28 all-black towns were founded in Oklahoma, all but four springing up in the old Indian Territory that became the eastern part of the state.

"A number of those—Redbird, Tallahassee, Boley, and Taft, for example—were satellite communities of Muskogee," noted cultural geographer Dr. George Carney in a 1985 interview. "By 1920, Muskogee had a thriving black commercial district of about 8,000, and a thriving black residential district as well. My theory is that when the satellite communities began to fail, many of the people moved to Muskogee, where the residential and business districts for blacks were already established."

Whatever the reasons, Muskogee reigns as one of the top towns in the country when it comes to producing notable jazz figures. As William W. Savage, Jr. notes in his book *Singing Cowboys and All That Jazz: A Short History of Popular Music in Oklahoma,* (University of Oklahoma Press, 1983), "It is remarkable that Jay McShann, Claude Williams, Samuel Aaron Bell, and Barney Kessel all were born in Muskogee. Theirs are names sufficiently prominent to secure that community's place in the history of American jazz, but they were not the only musicians the town produced."

Savage's supplemental list includes Walter and Joe Thomas, saxophone-playing brothers who worked with Jelly Roll Morton, among others. (Walter Thomas, nicknamed "Foots," spent several years as a player and arranger for Cab Calloway before leaving the performing side of the business in 1948 to become an agent and manager. His client list included fellow Muskogeean Bell.) Savage also cites saxophonist Don Byas, an Oklahoma City Blue Devil late in that band's run, and a Kansas City jazz figure before returning home to form a group at Langston University called Don Carlos and His Collegiate Ramblers (which is where he picked up "Don"—his real first name was Carlos). Later, Byas worked with the likes of Lionel Hampton, Duke Ellington and Dizzy Gillespie, and had a featured spot in the 1970 Newport Jazz

> "MOST OF OKLAHOMA'S JAZZMEN WERE BLACK MUSICIANS, AND MANY OF THESE BLACK JAZZMEN WERE FREEDMEN," EXPLAINED HISTORIAN LOGSDON. "THEY HAD THEIR ROOTS HERE BEFORE MUCH WHITE SETTLEMENT CAME IN. ALSO, THERE WAS TALK OF MAKING OKLAHOMA AN ALL-BLACK STATE IN THE 1890s AND 1900s, WHICH ATTRACTED A LOT OF BLACK PEOPLE."

Festival. Early on, he'd spent time in the band of still another Muskogee native, trumpeter T. (for Terrence) Holder, whose Dark Clouds of Joy and Twelve Clouds of Joy were two more progenitors of the Kansas City jazz sound.

Samuel Aaron Bell was well-known as a bassist with Duke Ellington's orchestra, but he also played with a number of other jazz greats—including fellow Okie Lester Young—and recorded several albums as a bandleader, where he was often billed simply as Aaron Bell. After receiving a doctorate degree from Columbia University, Bell became a professor of music at Essex County College in Newark, New Jersey, a position he held for many years beginning in 1970.

Claude Williams was a fiddler and guitarist who worked with the Dark Clouds of Joy in the 1930s (after Muskogeean T. Holder had turned the band over to another musician, Andy Kirk) and later with Basie's group. In the 1970s, he and Jay McShann began touring together, two major figures in the development of Kansas City jazz who both happened to be from the same Oklahoma town.

T. Holder isn't as well-known as most of the other Muskogee jazz cats. For one thing, his career wound down in the early 1940s. For another, his various Clouds of Joy operations were territory bands, just as the Blue Devils had been, seldom venturing outside the Southwest and Midwest and therefore not getting seen nor heard by audiences and critics on the coasts. Still, he was an influential figure to the young jazz players coming of age in the '30s, especially to Samuel Aaron Bell, as the bassist remembered in a 1985 conversation.

"A lot of the bands, the territory bands that used to tour, hit Muskogee on the way from Texas to Kansas City," he said. "T. Holder and the Clouds of Joy came through and played one time, and the bass player was late coming back from intermission. T. Holder hired me for that night, and later took my number and called me to play for him."

Similarly, McShann recalled how Clarence Love, during one of his Muskogee shows, "told me he might have to use me one night on the piano. That's when I got to thinkin' about this whole thing."

In the same 1985 conversation, McShann called saxophonist and bandleader Love "one of the old greats," and indeed, he was—even if the kind of music he played in Kansas City wasn't exactly Kansas City jazz.

"My hero was Guy Lombardo," said an octegenarian Love in 1990, puffing on his omnipresent cigar. "When I put together my orchestra, I put it together like Guy Lombardo's. I didn't play Kansas City music then, you know what I mean? I didn't play a black nightclub all the time I was in Kansas City. The only time I played for black people then was at private parties."

What he did do, however, was offer hungry jazz musicians of his acquaintance some chances to make a buck or two, even if they had to play music that was a little squarer than they liked. Several Blue Devils moonlighted in his Kansas City-based "sweet" band, including Lester Young and, for a brief time, Count Basie. Love was coy when asked about the persistent story that he let Basie go because the Count couldn't read music well enough.

"Now, the story's gotten out that I fired Basie," he responded with a smile. "The thing is, he wouldn't have gotten any satisfaction playing with my band. He played a different kind of music."

The music that Love and the rest of his African-American bands played in Kansas City was more appealing to white audiences, and that's who came to most of his gigs. In those days, segregation still reigned, and just as white and black audiences rarely mingled, neither did players, save for jam sessions that usually took place in the early hours of the morning, after most of the paying customers had found their respective ways home. Given Love's familiarity with both white audiences and black musicians, it makes sense that he went on to found Love's Lounge, Tulsa's first "black and tan" (that is, multiracial) nightclub, in the late 1940s.

A full decade before that, however, young white guitarist Barney Kessel was not only working with black bands in his Muskogee hometown, but also for mixed audiences, something that in retrospect seems positively revolutionary. To him, however, it was simply a way of learning more about the music he loved, and a logical extension of his friendship with Samuel Aaron Bell.

"I played with local white musicians in Muskogee, but I listened to blacks and ended up actually playing in their bands," Kessel said. "By keeping my eyes open and listening, I learned from them. I'd be playing tremolo and all this corny stuff, and they'd be trying to explain to me how to play different, how they'd heard it played in Kansas City.

"The thing was, in the late 1930s we'd play for dances, and both black and white would come. There was absolutely no social problem at all when I was playing with the black bands. We'd play the Grand Ballroom above the Grand Theatre on Second Street, a theater for blacks. Another place we'd play was the DeLuxe Ballroom, which was owned by a white couple. The night of a dance, the only white people in the building would be the two owners and me.

"I was 15 at the time," he added. "My mother was a little afraid, but when we were playing I never thought about it. There never was anything to be afraid of. Our common bond was our music."

As was the case with the Oklahoma City Blue

Devils, and would be the rule for Oklahoma groups down through the years—regardless of their musical styles—the jazz bands in Muskogee would produce some great players who'd go on to lasting national fame. Certainly, in those Depression-era days, there was competition among these outfits for the paying jobs available in town, as well as, in many of the players, a desire to be better than a weekend musician—to catch on in Kansas City and live the big-town jazz life. But even given that, there was a nurturing spirit at work in these people, a sense not only of obligation to their peers, but of a kind of paternal interest, especially on the part of the guys who'd been around. As Samuel Aaron Bell put it, "In those days in Muskogee, all the musicians were very friendly to us young musicians. They helped us, encouraged us, and they kept our ambition up."

"MY MOTHER WAS A LITTLE AFRAID, BUT WHEN WE WERE PLAYING I NEVER THOUGHT ABOUT IT. THERE NEVER WAS ANYTHING TO BE AFRAID OF. OUR COMMON BOND WAS OUR MUSIC."

2
CHAPTER TWO
THE OKLAHOMA CITY BLUE DEVILS — AND BEYOND

WOULD I like to go to Tulsa?
Boy, I sure would.
Let me off at Archer,
and I'll walk down to Greenwood

    —"Take Me Back to Tulsa" *by Bob Wills*

WE sat there in the car and listened, and after the show was over, I went behind the stage and introduced myself to the fiddler. He told me his name was Bob Wills. Of course, the name didn't mean anything to me. I just liked the way he played.

    —Herman Arnspiger, western-swing pioneer

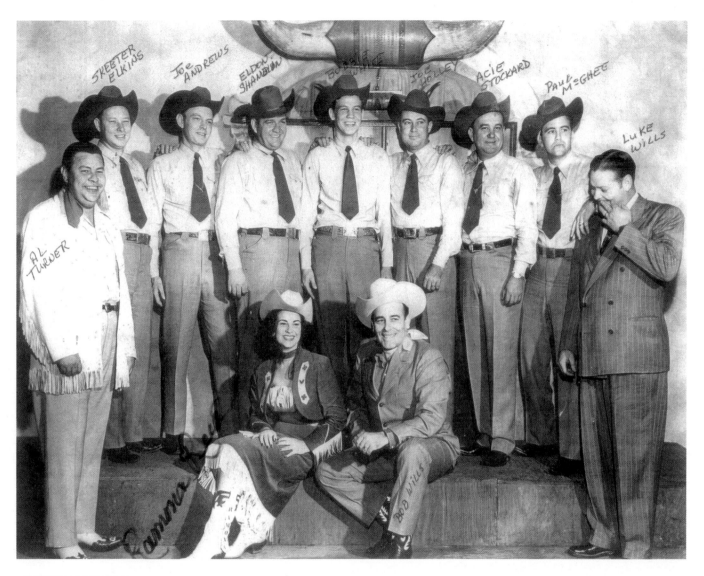

Bob Wills and his band early 1950s

As jazz is to Kansas City and New Orleans, and the blues are to Memphis, so is western swing to Tulsa. Born in Fort Worth, Texas, this danceable, jazzy, down-home music came to Oklahoma to grow up. The reason? It was a fiddling Lone Star expatriate named Bob Wills, who was virtually chased out of his home state by a vengeful ex-employer and ended up not only putting the final touches on this exciting new music in his adopted hometown, but also leading what was, for a time, the top-grossing dance band of any kind in the entire country.

The music Bob Wills honed and perfected in

Tulsa came from lots of places: the Texas ranch-house dances he'd played with his father as a youngster, where farmers and ranchers and their families would come from all over the area, roll up the rugs, and hit the floor until dawn; the African-American cotton pickers he worked side by side with on the hot and dusty Texas farms, soaking up the rhythms of their field hollers and the music they made in the cotton camps when the work day finally ended; and the carney-like, hustling atmosphere of the traveling medicine show, where an entertainer had to have plenty of novelty songs and snappy patter to hold the crowd and maybe sell a few boxes of candy until the medicine man took over with his own pitch.

Wills had done a little bit of a lot of things–including barbering, construction, family farming, and even some preaching–before the late '20s when he went on the road with an outfit called Doc's Medicine Show, doubling as both musician and a blackface comedian named Rastus. Minstrel shows featuring white entertainers who covered their faces with burnt cork or other skin-darkening agent and worked in dialect had begun in America in the middle 19th Century and peaked in popularity a few decades later. However, the blackface tradition continued to exert an influence on popular entertainment for a long time. For instance, *The Jazz Singer*, the 1927 Warner Brothers film considered Hollywood's first talking picture, famously features plenty of blackface entertainment from star Al Jolson. In the '20s, minstrel-show style entertainment was still so pervasive that some black entertainers of the time would slap on the blackface makeup themselves. That seems to have been the case with Billy King, the vaudevillian noted in our first chapter who was instrumental in the early life of the Oklahoma City Blue Devils.

Sources differ on whether it was 1928 or 1929 when Fort Worth resident Herman Arnspiger and a friend happened upon Doc's Medicine Show in an area of the city called the Riverside Addition. Arnspiger, in an interview conducted in September 1983 just a few months before his death, remembered the year as 1928, while Dr. Charles Townsend, in his superbly researched last word on Wills, *San Antonio Rose: The Life and*

"WILLS HAD DONE A LITTLE BIT OF A LOT OF THINGS–INCLUDING BARBERING, CONSTRUCTION, FAMILY FARMING, AND EVEN SOME PREACHING–BEFORE THE LATE '20S WHEN HE WENT ON THE ROAD WITH AN OUTFIT CALLED DOC'S MEDICINE SHOW, DOUBLING AS BOTH MUSICIAN AND A BLACKFACE COMEDIAN NAMED RASTUS."

Music of Bob Wills (University of Illinois Press, 1976) says it happened in 1929. Whichever year it was, this is how Arnspiger described his first glimpse of Bob Wills:

"We saw a crowd of people around a little ol' stage with a cover on it," he recalled. "It was a medicine show and a fiddle player was there playing in blackface."

As Arnspiger noted in the quote beginning this chapter, he waited and introduced himself to Wills after the show. A guitarist himself, Arnspiger was living behind a drugstore and he invited Wills to come over sometime and play. The next Sunday, Wills took him up on it.

"When he got there," Arnspiger recalled, laughing, "he wasn't in blackface. I almost didn't know the boy."

After an afternoon of jamming on the drugstore's front porch—a musical event that drew a sizable crowd—Wills asked Arnspiger to join the show. They both toured with the Doc for the next few months, until cold weather shut things down in December. Then they parted ways as they sought other work.

The next year, as the Great Depression tightened its merciless grip on the country, Arnspiger was out of his textile-mill job and scuffling to make some money playing music. "One day, I accidentally went by this drugstore, the same place where Bob and I had played the year before, walked in, and there sat Bob, drinking a Coca-Cola," Arnspiger remembered.

He knew that Fort Worth radio station KTAT was looking for a fiddler and guitarist for a new show, and suggested to Bob that they audition for it. As it turned out, Wills was only in town for a short time. He'd briefly stopped in Fort Worth with his family. They were all on the move, staying at a hotel on their way home from the eastern part of the state.

"He said, 'I can't do that,'" remembered Arnspiger. "'I'm with Daddy, Mama, and the kids, and we're headed back to west Texas to gather up crops.'"

Arnspiger, however, decided not to take no for an answer.

"Next morning at 4 a.m., I went over to beg and plead with Bob to stay. They had everything

"NEXT MORNING AT 4 A.M., I WENT OVER TO BEG AND PLEAD WITH BOB TO STAY. THEY HAD EVERYTHING LOADED IN THEIR TRUCK, READY TO GO BACK. I MUST'VE TALKED TO HIM UNTIL DAWN. FINALLY, UNCLE JOHN WILLS [BOB'S FATHER] HANDED HIM A COUPLE OF DOLLARS AND SAID, 'BOB, GO TRY OUT. IF YOU DON'T GET IT, USE THIS MONEY AND TAKE A BUS HOME.'"

loaded in their truck, ready to go back. I must've talked to him until dawn. Finally, Uncle John Wills [Bob's father] handed him a couple of dollars and said, 'Bob, go try out. If you don't get it, use this money and take a bus home.'"

Wills never had to use his dad's cash. The two got the gig at KTAT, a six-day-a-week morning show that allowed them to play dances at night. Writing in *San Antonio Rose*, Charles Townsend notes that the dance jobs they got were at events known as house parties, or house dances, and they were "really just country dances moved to town. They were very popular in the Southwest until Prohibition was repealed and dance halls and taverns became more plentiful."

During one of these house-dance jobs, they met a brash former cigar salesman named Milton Brown, who happened to be a first-rate vocalist. By that time, Wills and Arnspiger were using the name the Wills Fiddle Band, and Wills asked Brown to join. (Brown's guitar-playing 15-year-old brother, Durwood, was also told he could play with the group when he wasn't in school.)

In 1930, the Wills Fiddle Band–sans vocalist Brown, who wasn't needed on this particular job–entered a contest that would boost the group's fortunes. It was an "old fiddlers' contest" sponsored by another Fort Worth station, KFJZ. "We hadn't made much money to speak of up to that time," noted Arnspiger. "But the listeners voted us the best over a 12-week period and we won the contest."

First prize was a pair of fifty-dollar gold pieces, which, the guitarist said, "looked as big as dinner plates" to the two hardscrabble musicians. But the news wasn't all good. Because of the appearances on a rival station, the Wills Fiddle Band was bounced from KTAT. Naturally, the first place they looked for a new show was their recent benefactor, KFJZ.

The KFJZ program director was on vacation when Wills, Arnspiger and Brown arrived unannounced for an audition, sometime in the summer of 1930. So the group was instead auditioned by the station's staff pianist, a young fellow named Alton Stricklin. He'd later recall the incident in his book, *My Years with Bob Wills*, written with Jon McConal (The Naylor Company, 1976):

They looked like bad hombres. All needed shaves and Bob had his fiddle in a flour sack. I later learned that he had hocked it earlier for $5 and had borrowed it out of hock for this audition.

I introduced myself to them and they seemed nice. I learned that Wills would be playing the fiddle, Herman Arnspiger would be seconding on the guitar and Milton Brown would be the main vocalist.

"Boys, what kind of music do you play?" I asked.

"Different," said Wills. "The Wills Fiddle Band plays different."

He wasn't kidding. The trio's first selection was a wild number called "Who Broke the Lock on the Henhouse Door." Wrote Stricklin, "Milton sang with great gusto and Bob swung his fiddle wildly up and down, and all of the time just playing the hell out of it. Arnspiger was whacking and twirling and plunking his guitar like it was a piece of fire and he wanted to let it go but couldn't."

The music sounded downright bizarre to the young pianist; he figured they might be trying to be funny. But because the station was always in need of entertainment to chew up airtime—KFJZ didn't have any recorded-music programs yet—Stricklin put the Wills Fiddle Band on the air. That appearance, Stricklin wrote, netted several hundred letters and cards from enthusiastic listeners, and the group was hired to play six days a week. At the end of each week, they split fifteen bucks.

It wasn't long before the group left for a bigger Fort Worth station, WBAP, which put the men on the air as the Aladdin Laddies, sponsored by the Aladdin Lamp Company. By that time, noted *San Antonio Rose* author Townsend, other influences had found their way into the band's repertoire. "Old-time fiddle music was, of course, very popular in the WBAP listening area, and Wills played enough of it to satisfy this audience," he wrote. "But he had already borrowed enough from jazz and popular music to give his music a broader appeal and a swing that standard fiddle bands did not have..."

By January of 1931, the band had moved again, back to KFJZ, where they were working for an outfit called Burrus Mills, makers of Light Crust Flour. (In those days there was much more baking in American homes so flour companies were competitive and often heavily advertised.) As the Light Crust Doughboys, Wills, Arnspiger, and Brown—along with many other pioneers of the sound that would come to be known as western swing—would make their first real musical mark. Because of the mill's general manager—a fellow whose nickname of "Pappy" hinted at his autocratic nature—Bob Wills would flee Texas and land in Oklahoma, where he'd refine that sound into something not only unique, but immensely popular as well, using Tulsa's Cain's Ballroom as his base and clear-channel flamethrower KVOO to get into the homes and hearts and feet of people across a great big portion of this country, and beyond.

It was as much Bob's fault as it was Pappy's, I guess, because Pappy wanted everyone to be on the job every day, and to be there on time, and Bob wasn't there all the time when he thought he should be. They had their arguments. He'd fire Bob, and take him back, and so on, and so forth.

— *O. W. Mayo,* BOB WILLS' LONGTIME BUSINESS MANAGER

Wilbert Lee O'Daniel, known as W. Lee O'Daniel or simply as "Pappy," would eventually become a well-known Texas politician, his down-home style impressing voters enough to make him not only a governor, but a United States senator as well. In January of 1931, however, when Bob Wills made his first radio appearance as a Light Crust Doughboy, O'Daniel was the president and general manager of Burrus Mills, purveyors of Light Crust Flour. While Pappy didn't take to the music nor the musicians at first, he was eventually won over and became not only a fan but a contributor to the show—a situation that was probably a mixed blessing, considering that his close proximity to the daily program and its musicians ultimately led to conflicts between him and Bob Wills, the leader of the Doughboys.

By 1932, the broadcasts were a regional hit, having moved back over to WBAP, where they ultimately expanded into a number of other stations—even to Oklahoma City's KOMA—over the Southwest Quality Network (referred to in some sources as the Texas Quality Network). That was also the year that saw the resignation of Milton Brown. It happened after O'Daniel raised the musicians' pay, but told them at the same time they could no longer play dances. Brown and brother Durwood split, with Brown hiring some other good musicians and landing a spot on a rival station, where he promptly started booking dances. At the time of his 1936 death, Brown had already recorded over a hundred songs and was well on his way to a major career. Had he not died in an auto accident while taking a young woman home following one of his dance engagements, he might've rivaled Wills as the towering figure in western-swing music. Regardless of his

> "HAD HE NOT DIED IN AN AUTO ACCIDENT WHILE TAKING A YOUNG WOMAN HOME FOLLOWING ONE OF HIS DANCE ENGAGEMENTS, HE MIGHT'VE RIVALED WILLS AS THE TOWERING FIGURE IN WESTERN-SWING MUSIC."

relatively short life as a professional singer, he was hugely influential in its early development.

Back at Burrus Mills, O'Daniel insisted the musicians spend a 40-hour work week practicing and learning new tunes. (When they'd first started the program, O'Daniel had insisted they work full-time jobs at the mill. Wills had driven a truck, Arnspiger had worked on the loading docks, and Brown had been a salesman.) After auditioning dozens of singers, Wills hired the man who'd become his most popular and best-known vocalist during western swing's golden age. His name was Tommy Duncan, and Wills hired him after

O.W. Mayo

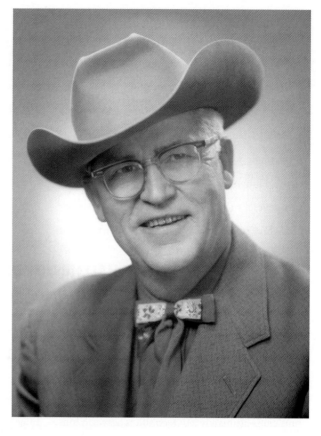

listening to him sing at a Forth Worth root beer stand. Duncan joined a Light Crust Doughboys that included recent additions Clifton "Sleepy" Johnston on tenor banjo (an important rhythm instrument in those pre-drum days) and Kermit Whalen on steel guitar and bass.

Things went along well enough for a year or so, although Brown's firing had exposed a rift between O'Daniel and Wills that grew wider and wider. Many reasons have been given for the final split. There was the fact that Brown was cleaning up in the dancehalls that were prohibited to Wills, making more money in one night—according to Charles Townsend—than Wills made for a whole week of radio broadcasts. For another, there was O'Daniel's resistance to Wills putting his brother Johnnie Lee, who was then driving a truck for the mill, to work in the band. According to the first book ever written about Bob Wills and the Texas Playboys, *Hubbin' It* (privately printed, 1938), the final straw had to do with Bob Wills and alcohol. It wasn't the first time that combination had led to trouble in Wills' life. It wouldn't be the last.

According to *Hubbin' It*'s author, *Tulsa Tribune* reporter Ruth Sheldon, it happened the day after beer was legalized in Texas, when "the whole town [of Fort Worth] was celebrating."

Bob and the boys took their instruments and wandered from beer tavern to beer tavern helping the rest of Ft. Worth drink up all the beer and playing wherever they went. O'Daniel, who had come to the conclusion that he and Bob could not work together any more, fired Bob for his part in the celebration and failure to appear for the following day's program.

The Light Crust Doughboys continued—they would, in fact, go on for decades—but they were now without not only Bob, but also Duncan and Whalen, both of whom vowed to stay with Wills.

Although the Light Crust Doughboys weren't allowed to play dances, O'Daniel would take them around Texas for personal appearances and special broadcasts from time to time. One of the towns they'd played was Waco, where a fireman named Bill Little had become a huge fan. After leaving the mill and O'Daniel, Wills drove to Waco, where he talked WACO station manager Everett Stover into giving the new band a radio show of its own. Then, he borrowed $25 from Little to get the rest of the boys to town.

As it turned out, Little's sister Cody was married to a man named O.W. Mayo. A white-collar oil-company man when he first saw Wills play, Mayo would become the business manager for both Bob and Johnnie Lee Wills, and one of the most important non-musicians in the development of western swing.

According to Townsend's *San Antonio Rose*, Wills began calling his band the Playboys after they came to radio station WACO. When Bill Little booked the group for a dance in downtown Waco, however, a newspaper ad for the event billed Wills' band under the older moniker of "Bob Wills' Fiddle Band," adding "(formerly Light Crust Doughboys)." By this time the group numbered five, with the addition of two band members' brothers: Johnnie Lee Wills on tenor banjo, and June Whalin, who'd been working in Fort Worth as a typewriter salesman, on rhythm guitar. They replaced Johnson and Arnspiger, respectively, who'd stayed at Burrus Mills.

According to Ruth Sheldon in *Hubbin' It*, the group's first try at a public dance didn't work out too well. "They played in an open air place on the outskirts of town and the heavy dew broke $36 worth of instrument strings. Five dollars was all they cleared at the gate, as the large crowd preferred to sit in automobiles listening to the music rather than to pay to dance."

The second one looked as though it was going

> **"THEY PLAYED IN AN OPEN AIR PLACE ON THE OUTSKIRTS OF TOWN AND THE HEAVY DEW BROKE $36 WORTH OF INSTRUMENT STRINGS. FIVE DOLLARS WAS ALL THEY CLEARED AT THE GATE, AS THE LARGE CROWD PREFERRED TO SIT IN AUTOMOBILES LISTENING TO THE MUSIC RATHER THAN TO PAY TO DANCE."**

to be better. But it, too, didn't end particularly well. As O.W. Mayo recalled in a 1986 interview:

My brother-in-law [Little] had booked them in the Woodmen Hall there in Waco, and he'd failed to take out a city permit, which was required. So the police came there and stopped the dance.

They'd been dancing for an hour or so. And my brother-in-law told them, 'If you'll not ask for your money back, why, we'll play another dance this next week, and those of you here tonight will get in free.'

The offer placated the crowd, which included Mayo himself, who'd stopped off to see the band. (His wife stayed in the car.) Something about the group got to him, and he found himself offering his help. He recalled:

I saw them and I saw they were sweating and so forth, and they didn't have any transportation. They had an old Buick that was just a wreck that they had borrowed from somebody in Fort Worth to get down there in.

My brother-in-law wanted to help them, but he was limited because the fire department had a rule that the firemen couldn't go outside and do other things. You know what I mean? Moonlight. So I said, "Bob, I'm marking time here for a while, and I know the territory pretty well, and if I can help you I'll be glad to."

He said, "I sure would appreciate it."

At the time, Mayo had just left the Cities Service Oil Company, where he'd worked for nine years, and he "had three different jobs I was dickering on, one with General Tire, one with American Oil, and one with Phillips Petroleum." His resume didn't include booking bands, but he quickly found out he had a knack for it.

That weekend, Miz Mayo and I went to a little community called Sharp, Texas, where her uncle lived. Miz Mayo's brother went with us. We went down to spend the night. We went through Cameron, Texas, and about six miles outside of Cameron, I saw a dance hall.

I stopped and asked the old boy, "Do you ever rent this?" He said, "'yeah.'" I said, "What do you rent it for?" He said, "'Five dollars, and I'll keep the concessions.'" I said, "I'll take it for next Saturday night."

Once in Sharp, Mayo also arranged for Bob Wills and the boys to play an afternoon show at the schoolhouse in that small town, preceding the dance in nearby Cameron. "Of course, everybody knew who Bob Wills was," Mayo pointed out, "because he'd been on the Doughboy show for so long. That's the only entertainment they had in those days—the radio."

Third time was the charm for the group. Mayo charged ten cents per person—"Mom, Dad, kids, whatever. If you had a family of five, you could bring 'em for fifty cents"—and after the school took its 25 percent cut, the band was left with thirty dollars. Then, they drove over to Cameron to play the dance, and got together for the split afterward. As Mayo remembered:

We'd rented a public-address system. We'd spent some money on placards and newspaper ads and so forth, and they paid me five dollars a day for my car. Divided six ways between the five of them and me, we had twenty-seven dollars and fifty cents apiece. Well, that was big money. Johnnie Lee had been making fifteen dollars a week driving that truck [for Burrus Mills]. Since Bob was the head man, they had been giving him thirty-five dollars a week at Burrus Mills, but Tommy Duncan and Kermit had been making eighteen dollars a week as sidemen.

So we all had twenty-seven dollars and fifty cents, which was a lot of money. They bought 'em some new strings, had their shirts laundered, and in a week's time, I had them playing somewhere every night.

As that financial breakdown indicates, the Playboys, or former Light Crust Doughboys, or the Bob Wills Fiddle Band—whatever they might be called on handbills and in newspaper advertising for a particular gig—had become a commonwealth band, dividing the profits equally. No longer was Bob Wills paid more for being the bandleader. Once freed from the restrictions of the mill and Pappy O'Daniel, including the pay scale, these men reverted to the all-for-one and one-for-all approach of the Oklahoma City Blue Devils, sharing what they made in equal portions.

No, the Oklahoma City Blue Devils weren't the first commonwealth band, and far from the only one. And yes, there were and are commonwealth groups from every part of the country. But again, it's worthwhile to consider the strong spirit of brotherhood and emphasis on taking care of the other guy that typifies so many Oklahoma musical acts. Looking at the state and its musicians in that light, it seems only right that Bob Wills and his Playboys soon headed for the Sooner State—where they, and the music that would come to be known as western swing, would reach full and brilliant flower.

The station in Waco they were on was just a small station. If you got over 50 or 60 miles away, you didn't hear it. But his popularity had gone on because he had been on the Texas Quality Network for Burrus Mills, and that included WFAA Fort Worth, WOAI San Antonio and KBRC Houston—three big stations. Bob was a showman, and I knew that the people who were coming were eating it up, enjoying the music, and I saw the potential. So Bob and I came to Oklahoma City.

— *O. W. Mayo*

"Mayo, of course I want you to go with me," Bob said. "But if you or any of the other boys don't want to go you can stay. I'm leavin'. I'm goin' places and nothin' can stop me. This is a little old hundred-watt radio station here and folks outside of 20 miles away

can't hear us. The cotton money is all gone. It's goin' to be tough country to live in until next fall. I'm goin' someplace where everybody can know me and I'm goin' to the top."

— Bob Wills, QUOTED IN *Hubbin' It*

Time and conflicting memories have obscured the specific reasons why Bob Wills decided to pack up and move his band across the Red River, and just who in the band thought it was a good idea and who didn't. But surely the flight north had a lot—probably *mostly*—to do with Bob's old boss Pappy O'Daniel. Saddled with the task of maintaining a Light Crust Doughboys band without its popular leader, O'Daniel apparently first tried to win Bob back by intimidation, filing a $10,000 damage suit against the new Wills band for using the term "formerly Light Crust Doughboys" in its advertising. When the case was dismissed at the district level, O'Daniel, on behalf of Burrus Mills, appealed to a higher court. Apparently, old Pappy figured to sue Wills back into the fold.

"He wanted Bob back because he realized after Bob left that no one could take Bob Wills' place," Mayo told Charles R. Townsend. "They didn't have the popularity and pull."

After an appeal and a petition for a rehearing, both at O'Daniel's request, the whole thing finally ground to a halt in late September of 1935. Although the legal costs had left Wills and the band strapped, by that time they were firmly entrenched in Tulsa, Oklahoma, where a couple of major sections of the Texas Playboys story had already fallen into place: the Cain's Ballroom and radio station KVOO. One would become, as the famous western-swing revivalist Ray Benson has called it, the Carnegie Hall of western swing. The other would use its 25,000 (later 50,000) watts of power to blast the Playboys' music throughout the Southwest and beyond.

In fact, though, their first Oklahoma broadcasts weren't made over KVOO at all. Instead, they first hit the airwaves over another legendary radio station, Oklahoma City's KOMA. Mayo explained it this way:

We wanted to go on KOMA in Oklahoma City, because Burrus Mills had been piping a [Light Crust Doughboys] show there for quite a while—they used telephone lines, you know, to do remote shows—and Bob and the Doughboys were well known. So we approached the manager and he said, "Bob, you know I'd love to have you, but I can't hire you. I'd lose that account with O'Daniel, with Burrus Mills." In other words, he didn't want to gamble against something that he had already. The Light Crust Doughboys were still going. He [O'Daniel] had brought in musicians, and the show went on. It wasn't the same show, but the show went on.

So we went over to WKY, and they told us "fine."

We told them when we'd be there, and I went on up a week ahead, and got out and booked a date in El Reno and Chickasha, I believe it was, and one in a club in Oklahoma City. The band came up, and we went on the air over WKY.

We were on the air just about a week, and one morning, Daryl McAllister, the program director, called me and said, "I want to see you and Bob in the studio."

When they got there, McAllister told them that W. Lee O'Daniel had called the station manager—"the big shot," Mayo termed him—and said he'd been thinking seriously about moving the Light Crust Doughboys show from KOMA to WKY. But now, since WKY had seen fit to put Bob Wills on the air, O'Daniel figured he'd just leave the Light Crust Doughboys on KOMA. Said Mayo:

He gave him such a talk that he thought all he had to do was kick Bob off the station and he'd have the Light Crust Doughboys show. I said, "Let us talk to him," but Daryl wouldn't. You couldn't talk to the manager of the station. Daryl said, "I'll tell you what. There's a new station that's opened in Tulsa, and I think they'd be tickled to death to have you." It had opened in January, and this was February [1934]. That was KTUL—but it was a small station. He said, "I'll tell you what I'll do. I know the manager of the station, and I'll call him." So he talked to Gillespie, and Gillespie said, "Yeah. Send 'em on over."

Leaving the rest of the boys in Oklahoma City, Mayo and Wills drove to Tulsa to check out the new station. With them was Everett Stover, the former WACO station manager—who also happened to be a trumpeter. "He'd been on the show with Bob and did all the announcing while we were there," Mayo said, "and Everett thought enough of it that he quit his job at WACO to come with us. He saw the possibilities, because he knew about the fan mail and all."

Then, somewhere along the way, Mayo came up with an idea that, literally, changed the course of western-swing music.

On our way over, I said, "Bob, KVOO radio is over there, and they're a 25,000-watt station. This station we're going to is only a 500-watt station. Let's go see KVOO first, and we might get a chance to get on that station."

So we got to Tulsa, and we went down First Street, got a shave at the barber shop, got cleaned up, and went to KVOO.

The station manager, William B. Way, wasn't in when they called, but the three impressed the receptionist enough about the urgency of their visit that she soon located him. With a chuckle, Mayo recalled what happened once Way arrived:

We gave him a song and dance, and directly Way stopped us and said, "Yeah, I know.

You're the hottest stuff on the market." Laughed, you know. He said, "Where's the band?"

I said, "Oklahoma City."

He said, "There's the phone."

So I picked up the phone and called 'em, and they got here about dusk, I guess. Way said, "I'm going to put you on the air tonight at twelve midnight. That'll be a good audience for you, and we'll see what they think of you."

When they put us on the air, we were down in the basement of the old Wright Building, right behind the [downtown] post office. So we went on the air at twelve midnight and said we'd give a picture of the band to the one who sent a letter or card from the furthest distance. That winning card or letter came from Oakland, California. We were clear channel, and they didn't have all these little stations going, so we didn't have much interference.

That, of course, was much of the key to the explosion of Bob Wills' music across the southwestern part of the country, and beyond, in the mid-to-late 1930s. In those pre-FM days, a powerful AM station like KVOO (whose call letters stood, aptly enough, for Voice Of Oklahoma) could cover a great deal of territory, especially when there were no other stations for hundreds of miles that shared the same frequency. KVOO was, to use a bit of radio-biz slang, a clear-channel flamethrower, whose programs could be heard in cities, and even states, far beyond Tulsa's city limits.

By the time Wills and the Playboys made their first broadcast, KVOO was already known for its music programming. Perhaps the most famous pre-Wills band on the station was an outfit called Otto Gray and His Oklahoma Cowboys, which some have cited as the first commercial western band in America. As writer Carla Chlouber put it in the winter 1997-98 edition of the *The Chronicles of Oklahoma*, a historical periodical, "...they were the first nationally known group to play western music, wear cowboy clothing, and perform before a wide audience, both on stage and over the radio." Like the Wills band a decade later, KVOO helped popularize Gray's aggregation by getting its music into homes across a good part of the country. Cowboy movie and singing star Gene Autry would also get a career boost at KVOO, as would newscaster Paul Harvey, while multiple award-winning disc jockey and country-music recording artist Billy Parker would find a longtime home on the station, his voice becoming synonymous with the Voice Of Oklahoma.

Officially beginning its run in 1925, KVOO hung in there for nearly eight decades as a powerful purveyor of music for much of America, surviving the FM blitz until 2002, when, under new ownership, it transmogrified into a right-wing talk outlet. An FM version of KVOO, however, featuring a country-music format, still exists at this writing.

Wills and the Playboys made their first KVOO broadcast just as February 10, 1934, dawned. For the next few weeks, they were all over the place at the station, showing up on morning, afternoon, and evening shows—all "sustaining" broadcasts, which meant that the musicians didn't get paid by the station. But, noted Mayo, while they weren't getting any money for being on KVOO, the ability to reach all those people soon began to pay off.

We'd just tell 'em we were available for dance engagements and schools and so forth, and pretty soon the letters began to come in, and the calls came in, and in a week's time we were playing every night. We'd be going to play a dance, and we'd stop and play a program at school. Anything. And people would stop and eat with us—that's the way it was.

That kind of rapport and identification with their audiences, while undeniably something that helped Bob and the Playboys get more bookings, was also born out of the spirit that emerged during the Great Depression, which was raging across the country at the time. It was a spirit of sharing and cooperation and acceptance that found a special manifestation in the Dust Bowl, where helping a neighbor out could literally mean the difference between life and death. Live music may not have held the same sort of importance when it came to survival of the body, but it was a necessary thing for the survival of the spirit. Wills and his people instinctively knew that suffering people needed *something* to alleviate their misery and buoy their spirits, if only for a while.

"In those days, that's all they *had*," said Mayo of the music. "It was the Depression days. And we didn't hold anybody up. We'd charge forty cents or fifty cents, maybe seventy-five cents or a dollar for a couple."

At first, the band began playing its local dances at the Pla-Mor, a second-story venue built over a garage. The Tulsa events were scheduled for Thursday nights, with the weekends devoted to out-of-town dates. "About eighty or ninety percent of our engagements were for civic, fraternal, or patriotic organizations," noted Mayo. "We found that by doing that we were playing for reputable sponsors. You know what I mean? We weren't playing in any clubs or dives.

"Then, too, there was a federal amusement tax that could be charged [on tickets] above forty cents, and the veterans' places could get a permit to waive the federal tax as long as it was a benefit." He chuckled. "We learned a lot of tricks."

While Mayo was learning the "tricks" of booking a band, Wills continued to experiment with the sound and size of his outfit, which had become known as the Texas Playboys. His laboratory would turn out to be a building called Cain's Dancing Academy—which, as the Cain's Ballroom, would soon become known as the Home of Bob Wills, a designation that continues to this day.

Ol' Daddy Cain, he'd never had anything but a modern type of music [in Cain's Dancing Academy], because he was teaching ballroom dancing, waltzing and foxtrots and what have you, and he built his dance audience from his dance classes and vice versa. What played regular was about a five-piece sax, drum and clarinet, you know, a little small combo. That's the type of music that he played. But when we played that dance that night, we saw the crowd that we'd draw, and it opened our eyes about the possibilities.

— *O.W. Mayo*

On New Year's Night 1935, Bob Wills and the Texas Playboys first played the Cain's Dancing Academy. It was the kind of gig Mayo liked to book—a benefit show for the nurses' association at Tulsa's Morningside Hospital. They got $100 for the engagement. They also got a new Tulsa home.

Madison "Daddy" Cain leased the building that bore his name, but because he'd had a stroke the year before, his dancing-academy classes were being run by a fellow named Howard Turner. The Cain's was about twice the size of the Pla-Mor, and the nurses' show proved to Mayo and Wills that the band could draw enough people to fill it. They struck a deal with Cain and Turner, moved the band's local dance headquarters from the Pla-Mor, and began playing at the Cain's.

As all that was going on, Bob Wills was working on the sound of the Texas Playboys, replacing musicians who left and adding a few as he went along. It must've galled his old nemesis Pappy O'Daniel—who'd tried and failed to get Wills pulled from KVOO using some of the same tactics that had worked at WKY—when Bob rehired Herman Arnspiger and took on a teenage steel guitarist named Leon McAuliffe, both of whom had been with O'Daniel's Light Crust Doughboys. McAuliffe and his "Steel Guitar Rag" would help usher in the use of that instrument in pop music (as well as introduce the phrase "Take it away, Leon," into the American vernacular.) As McAuliffe told *San Antonio Rose* author Townsend about the use of the steel guitar in Wills' fiddle-based dance outfit, "It was another thing we pioneered in Bob's band. Bob wanted to be a first at everything. And he wanted to create."

While Wills wasn't the first bandleader to use a steel guitarist in music intended for dancing, he and McAuliffe surely did much to popularize the concept. Bob hired the young steel player in 1935, the same year he added another musician to the Texas Playboys—one who, indeed, was a first.

In 2001, during the celebration of his 90th birthday in his hometown of Rogers, Arkansas, drummer William "Smokey" Dacus recalled how he became the first drummer in what was then called "hillbilly" music.

I was playing in a hotel band, but I liked Dixieland. Of course, I couldn't play Dixieland at the hotel, but afterwards I'd go out to a place outside of Tulsa—I forget the name of it—and I'd play what I wanted to, just for kicks. We'd play 'til daylight, playing for a kitty, and some drunk'd always come up and ask us to play 'Wearin' of the Green' or something.

So Bob was hunting for a drummer, and he came out and saw me. When he asked me to join him, I thought he'd lost his mind. I said, "What the hell do you want with a drummer in a fiddle band?" He stuck that big cigar in his mouth, and poked me in the chest, and he said, "Because I want to take your kind of music and my kind of music—and make it all swing." He broke the ice, as far as having a drummer in a country band. But for four or five years after that, I was the only one.

Before Dacus, the fiddle-based dance bands of the Southwest used bass and often tenor banjo—which Johnnie Lee Wills played in the Playboys—as their rhythm instruments. After Dacus came along, the group kept Johnnie Lee on tenor banjo, but strengthened the beat and danceability with a drummer. The use of a drummer in a dance band seems obvious to us now; then, it was revolutionary.

The true development of what would become western swing began with Wills handpicking the men he wanted to help him create this new sound, based in fiddle music but already becoming a great deal more. The summer of 1935 found Wills making a sojourn to his old Fort Worth stomping grounds, where he sought out an old acquaintance. Alton Stricklin was the KFJZ staff pianist who'd given the scruffy trio calling itself the Bob Wills Fiddle Band an audition and radio show a few years earlier. It was Wills' turn to reciprocate.

In his book *My Years with Bob Wills*, Stricklin recalled a particular summer night in 1935. At the time, he was playing in a Texas nightspot with a group called the Hi Flyers, getting ready to go back to his day job of teaching school. Then, Bob Wills strolled into the place.

He was wearing expensive cowboy boots. He had on an expensive and tailored western suit. His pants were tucked inside his boots and he was wearing spurs. He had on a little black tie with a large diamond stick-pin in it. And he had on a big white western hat. He was tall and straight. He walked up to me and said, "Hi, Mr. Stricklin."

"Are you Bob Wills?" I asked.

He kinda grinned and said he was. I was impressed. And, shocked. He didn't look like the Bob Wills I had known who had played "Who Broke the Lock on the Henhouse Door" those three years ago.

As Stricklin remembered it, Wills told him,

"Strick, I've hit it pretty big up in Tulsa. I've got a radio program and it's going pretty good. We're making about $2000 a week." To Stricklin, who was making $3 on Wednesday nights and $5 on Fridays as the piano player for the Hi Flyers, that figure must've seemed astronomical. Then, Wills told him about the piano situation with the Texas Playboys. Recalled Stricklin:

> [Wills said] "I got an old boy who sings. His name is Tommy Duncan. He also plays the piano, but he doesn't know too much about it. He gets a lot of laughs but I'm looking for a better piano player. I'm going to need one in September."
>
> "Are you offering me a job?" I asked.
>
> "Yeah, I am," he said.
>
> "How much does it pay?" I asked
>
> "Thirty bucks," said Wills.
>
> "A month?" I asked.
>
> "No, a week," he replied.

The reason Wills needed a piano player so quickly was that the band had its first recording session coming up in Dallas. Obviously, it was an important opportunity for the band, one that could—and would—take the Playboys to another level, and Wills knew that the group needed a much stronger instrumentalist than Duncan—who, it's been said, wrecked almost as many pianos as he played. "Now, old Tommy knows a few chords and he's been doing his stuff at the dances," Stricklin remembered Wills saying. "But we are going to make some recordings in September and we need a piano player who can play some breaks and chords that will be acceptable to the recording people."

For his part, Stricklin told Wills, simply, "This is the greatest thing that ever happened to me." For years afterward, he would be known as Brother Al Stricklin, Bob Wills' first and most famous piano player.

We have fun because Bob taught us to have fun. He was so unpredictable that in all those years, it never did get dull.

— *Eldon Shamblin,* LEGENDARY GUITARIST AND ARRANGER

That first Texas Playboys session in Dallas, packed into that busy Playboys year of 1935, put onto shellac such Wills classics as "Maiden's Prayer," "Osage Stomp" and "Four or Five Times." Some of the cuts featured horns—trombone and saxophone—along with the rest of the instrumentation. By the time of the Playboys' second session in Chicago the next year, Everett Stover had added his trumpet to the mix. And in the early 1940s, when Wills led a large western-swing band that some say was every bit the musical equal of the mainstream swing bands of the Big Band Era, he took a group into the studio that included two brass and three reed players.

By then, his addition of guitarist and arranger

Eldon Shamblin to the band was paying off as well. Tulsa native Shamblin had been with another KVOO group, Dave Edwards and His Alabama Boys, before joining Wills in 1937. He stayed with Wills in some capacity for almost a quarter of a century, an important component of the Bob Wills sound, and of western-swing music itself. Many years later, Rolling Stone called him the best rhythm guitarist in the world. In a 1985 conversation, Shamblin recalled why he started playing the instrument that would make him famous.

When I was with the Alabama Boys, I was a singer, but I hated singing so bad that I picked up the guitar because I knew I was going to have to do something else. I'd played a little rhythm guitar before that, but when I came to Tulsa [from a radio show in Oklahoma City] it was singing that got me the job.

After I got to Tulsa, I tried to learn to play enough guitar so I wouldn't have to learn how to sing. It's funny how things work out, isn't it?

Bob Wills, on the other hand, was a fiddle player who liked to sing, at least occasionally. Tommy Duncan was, from his hiring, the group's primary vocalist—an analogue to Frank Sinatra with the Tommy Dorsey Orchestra and Ray Eberle with the Glenn Miller Orchestra. But Wills liked to spread the vocals around a little, with musicians like McAuliffe, fiddler Jesse Ashlock and bassist Joe Frank Ferguson getting the occasional nod, along with Wills himself, who always sang at least one or two selections on virtually every recording session. One of his particular favorites was "Rosetta," the ballad co-written and popularized by jazz figure Earl "Fatha" Hines. Wills not only sang it innumerable times on stage and in the recording studio; he also gave the name to one of his daughters.

A close listen to Wills' vocalizing—on just about any of his numbers, but especially on "Rosetta"—reveals an interesting fact. In musicians' parlance, Wills "broke meter," giving odd line readings of lyrics, with different emphasis and pacing from the original. To someone paid to keep the rhythm correct, like Smoky Dacus, a vocalist who broke meter—even if it was his boss—was galling. As Dacus recalled:

"Rosetta" was simple. The song had 32 beats. But when Bob did it, it was sometimes 30 beats, sometimes 34, sometimes 30 and a half. I'd tell him about it, and he'd say, "I don't give a damn how many beats it has. If it doesn't feel right, it's not right."

I remember when he first learned the song. I had a record of Fatha Hines' "Rosetta," and I took it out to Bob's house. He was living in a two-story building at Second and Peoria [in Tulsa], and there was a little flat-roofed grocery store right across the street. I took the record in and he listened to it and learned the words, and as soon as he started singing it he started breaking the rhythm. I listened to him awhile, and then I went and got the record

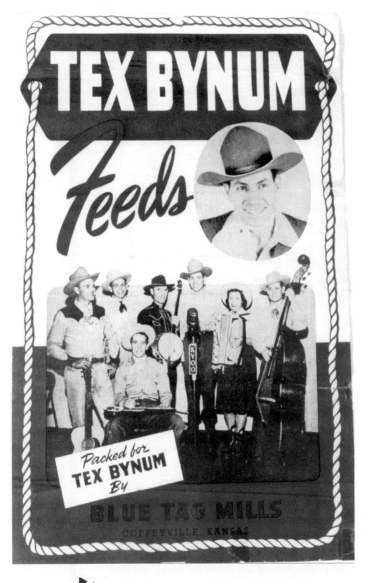

Tex Bynum and his band

off the machine. I said, "Bob, you've got a license to do anything you want, but you don't have any license to butcher."

Laughing, Dacus continued. "So I went out on his porch, and I took that 78, and I sailed it—and it landed on the roof of that grocery store. As far as I know, it's still there."

Wills may not have had the best sense of timing as a singer, but you couldn't touch him when it came to talking on a record. Virtually every Wills recording—with a few notable exceptions—features snippets of commentary from the bandleader, hearkening back to the smart-aleck comedy patter of his minstrel-show days. Even given all the other musical innovations introduced or popularized by Wills—the use of steel guitar and drums, the horn section, the melding of influences that took the traditional Southwestern fiddle band and turned it into something wholly other—it's the chirpy "ah-*Has*" and often-comic introductions of soloing sidemen that, as much as anything else, define Bob Wills' music to this day. And just as other bands throughout the country—especially in the West and Southwest—would appropriate Wills' inventive mix of styles and instrumentation, other bandleaders would also adopt his particular way of introducing sidemen and livening things up with muttered asides. Front men like Nebraska's Ole Rasmussen and Texas' Hoyle Nix, to name two of the more obvious ones, aped Wills' patter so perfectly that they often sounded like straight-ahead impersonators.

To many, especially during his peak years of the late '30s and early '40s, Bob Wills was what

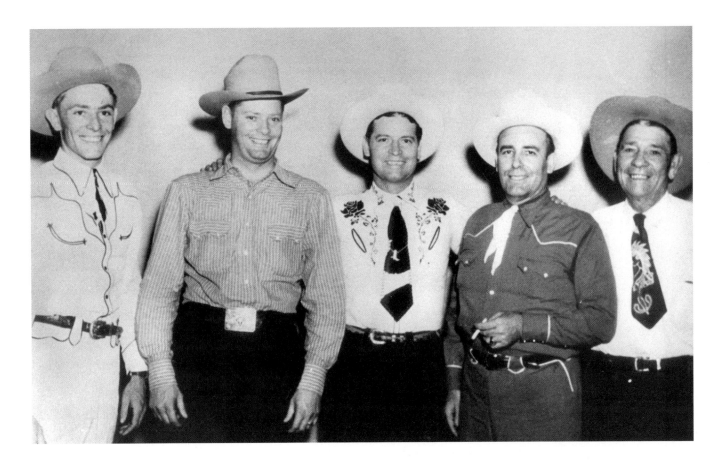

from left, Billy Jack Wills, Luke Wills, Johnnie Lee Wills, Bob Wills and their father, "Uncle John" Wills, late 1940s

Elvis Presley would become in the 1950s—a larger-than-life figure from humble, rural beginnings, who soared into the pop-culture stratosphere and achieved near-mythic status, yet somehow always kept that connection to the working classes. Bob Wills was the Elvis of his time, a man who—as saxophonist Glenn "Blub" Rhees once noted—could turn an ordinary band into something special simply by walking onto the stage. Like Elvis, his imitators were legion. And like the rockabilly music that Presley popularized, western swing also attracted a number of practitioners who brought something different to the mix, taking the Tulsa-based Wills sound and putting their own spin on it, helping it grow and flourish. Not surprisingly, a disproportionate number of them were solidly rooted in Oklahoma soil.

We had real good turnouts then. I had my own following and we'd get the overflow from the Cain's. We didn't carry as many musicians as Bob Wills did, but we played a lot of the same style and the same numbers as Bob.

—*Tex Bynum,* BANDLEADER

We came here [to Tulsa] in '34, and in '42 Bob went into the service. When he got out of the service in '43, he went out to California, and he stayed out in California. He came back here for one year in '58, and then he left. But Johnnie Lee was here all that period of time. Johnnie Lee took over when Bob left, you see, and as far as the length of the time and all our operations here and so forth, Johnnie Lee was involved much longer than Bob. But Bob would come back for anniversaries, and engagements, and this, that, and the other. He was still a part of the family, if you know what I mean.

—O.W. Mayo,

BUSINESS MANAGER FOR BOB AND JOHNNIE LEE WILLS

I was 17 when I did my first show with Bob's band. I played tenor banjo. As a matter of fact, I signed my first Social Security card in the office of Cain's Academy.

—Luther J. "Luke" Wills

I have nothing but the finest memories of the Cain's. I grew up there.

—Billy Jack Wills

When it came to western swing music, there were others, and there were the brothers—Johnnie Lee, Luther J. and Billy Jack, Bob Wills' three younger brothers. Second brother Johnnie Lee, of course, had been at Burrus Mill with Bob, and by the time the Playboys crossed the Red River for good in 1934, he was already established as the band's tenor-banjo player. Four years later, Bob sent him out on his own as the leader of a group called the Rhythmairs, a kind of satellite group spun off the Texas Playboys. The Rhythmairs didn't last very long, but Johnnie Lee and the idea of auxiliary Wills groups did. After Bob left Tulsa, Johnnie Lee Wills and the group variously called All the Boys, All His Boys, or simply the Boys—the "boys" including some of the same personnel who'd been in the Playboys—jumped into the void that was left, never missing a beat, playing the dances and doing the KVOO broadcasts just as Bob had done. And while the band may not have had the national stardom Johnnie Lee's older brother enjoyed, it did all right, with a couple of big hit singles ("Rag Mop" and "Peter Cottontail") and a regional show sponsored, for a time, by General Mills.

The other two brothers also ended up leading their own bands. Third brother Luther J. "Luke" Wills had the Rhythm Busters, a group that held forth for stretches in an important western-swing venue about a hundred miles down the road from the Cain's, Oklahoma City's Trianon Ballroom (where, for a short time in the late '40s, Bob himself set up shop) as well as in California. Youngest brother Billy Jack Wills and His Western Swing Band was a first-class small outfit that took over the Wills Point nightspot in Sacramento, California—

which belonged to oldest brother Bob—in the early '50s. Luke was a bassist, Billy Jack a bassist and drummer, although in their own bands they were primarily front men and occasional vocalists. Just like brother Johnnie Lee, both did some major-label recording, although neither had a hit. Billy Jack, however, had a hand in writing two of the Texas Playboys' most famous tunes: "Faded Love" (designated Oklahoma's official "Country & Western Song" many years later by the state legislature) and "Lily Dale."

When musicians got hired for one of the Wills bands in the '40s, they weren't just joining a specific outfit. Instead, they were signing on with an organization, one with important units on the West Coast as well as in Tulsa. And, while some longtime Wills sidemen stayed in one place for most of their tenure—pianist Clarence Cagle and fiddler Curly Lewis, both linchpins of Johnnie Lee's band in Tulsa, come immediately to mind—many traveled back and forth between bands and states, going wherever they were needed—or, more specifically, wherever Bob needed them. Among the people Bob Wills moved into and out of his bands were his brothers themselves. Before and after their bandleading days, both Billy Jack and Luke played with the Texas Playboys and Johnnie Lee Wills' Boys as well. In a 1982 interview, Billy Jack recalled how, as a teenager, he'd "go down to the Cain's and watch Bob or Johnnie Lee and just itch to get up on that bandstand myself." Because an eye problem kept him from getting drafted into World War II, he was able to scratch that itch before he was out of his teens. By that time, his brother Luke had been playing, first with Bob and then with Johnnie Lee, for several years. Except for his tenure as the leader of the Rhythm Busters, Luke stuck with the Texas Playboys and Johnnie Lee's band, not only recording and touring but becoming a presence on the radio as well.

Bob and Johnnie Lee Wills' noontime radio broadcasts over KVOO have become the stuff of legend, especially around the Tulsa area, since the broadcasts didn't reach as far in the daytime as they did at night. Old-timers tell stories of farmers and ranchers coming in from the fields at lunchtime and hooking their radios up to a precious battery in order to hear the show. City folks of the time remember how a person could walk down a Tulsa street in the summer, when windows were open, and not miss a note of Wills music, because every radio was tuned to the program. The noon broadcasts were so successful that for a short time around 1940, KVOO also had a morning show featuring a Wills band.

There wasn't a lot of preparation time for any of these live shows, which sometimes led to humorous, awkward, or embarrassing moments. In a 1994 interview, Luke Wills remembered one particular incident involving O.W. Mayo, who was an announcer as well as the Wills brothers' business manager, and the accomplished jazz-influenced fiddler Jesse Ashlock, a good friend of Luke's who, as Luke recalled, "was a pretty big kidder."

One morning, we were getting ready to do a hymn. How it worked was that Mr. Mayo would do a commercial and then he'd announce our next song. Well, our sponsor was [the laxative] Black Draught, and when Mr. Mayo finished the commercial and announced our hymn number, nobody but Jesse made the connection. He got tickled, and then Mr. Mayo got tickled, but you couldn't laugh when you were doing a sacred number, you know.

The hymn was "I Shall Not be Moved," and we sure had a tough time getting through it.

Steel-guitarist Leon McAuliffe wasn't a Wills family member, but he was the next closest thing. Coming to the Playboys as a teenager in 1935, he'd been one of the important early musicians who'd helped Wills launch his new sound. He'd stayed with the Playboys, occasionally singing and composing as well as playing, until 1942, when he enlisted in the Navy. McAuliffe eventually led the official Bob Wills tribute band—Bob Wills' Original Texas Playboys—after Wills' death in 1975.

In between, he led his own western-swing outfit, Leon McAuliffe and the Cimarron Boys. Based in Tulsa's Cimarron Ballroom for much of its life, both the group and the venue had a good run, becoming the town's major competition for Johnnie Lee Wills and the Cain's Ballroom. McAuliffe even had his own show on KVOO.

After leaving the service and organizing his own band in Tulsa, McAuliffe pursued—at least initially—a different sound. It was, if you will, a style that emphasized the "swing" over the "western," an approach much less countrified than that of his former boss. This probably had a lot to do with his time in the service, when, as a flight instructor at an air base in Norman, Oklahoma, he'd met and befriended Tex Beneke, the famed Glenn Miller Orchestra alumnus who was conducting a military band on the base at the time. They began playing together, and McAuliffe became convinced that straight swing and jazzy pop music was what he wanted to do.

Indeed, when he got back to Tulsa that's exactly what he did. But according to saxophonist Bob Herrick, who played with McAuliffe in the late '40s, he nearly starved doing it. As Herrick explained in a 2005 interview, McAuliffe's outfit had been playing at a popular Tulsa nightspot called the Blue Moon in 1946 with his "contemporary band," where it was doing good business—probably because the Blue Moon often featured straight swing and dance outfits. But after the open-air nightspot finished its season, McAuliffe had to take the group out on the road because, as Herrick explained, "There was no place in Tulsa big enough to support that band." And the places he got booked were usually the places he'd played as a member of Bob Wills' Texas Playboys, where the phrase "Take It Away, Leon" still meant swing of the western variety.

In a 1977 interview with the *Tulsa Tribune's* Jim Downing, McAuliffe himself told what happened next. "[I]n those places," he said, "people would come up to the stand and ask, 'Where are your fiddles? Why don't you play 'San Antonio Rose' and 'Steel Guitar Rag' like you used to?' I'd have a big crowd the first time out, but it kept dropping off and finally I didn't have any crowds at all."

Noted Herrick, "We'd go back to those places, and the crowd would be cut in half each time. We might get 600 the first time, and then 300 the second, and 150 the third. It didn't work. People couldn't dance to that music. He lost the equivalent of $50,000 or $60,000 before he went back to western music."

Within a year after reverting to a sound more like the classic Wills style he'd helped create, McAuliffe had enough money to buy Tulsa's Akdar Temple building and convert it to a dancehall, the Cimarron Ballroom. Interestingly enough, according to Herrick, it was the great Wills guitarist Eldon Shamblin—then playing with McAuliffe between stints with the Texas Playboys—who finally convinced "Take It Away, Leon" to return to western swing.

Although he may not be as well-remembered by Tulsans as Johnnie Lee Wills and Leon McAuliffe, there was a third top-tier bandleader in town in those post-World War II days, and just as McAuliffe had emphasized the "swing" part of the music, Art Davis and His Rhythm Riders leaned toward the "western" side.

It was only natural. An accomplished fiddler, Davis had played with several early western-swing bands in his native Texas, including Milton Brown's Musical Brownies, Roy Newman and His Boys, Bill Boyd's Cowboy Ramblers and even the Light Crust Doughboys. But by the time he set up shop in Tulsa, his "western" credentials were impeccable, since he had spent the late '30s and early '40s working in cowboy pictures in Hollywood. He'd even starred in a half-dozen westerns with his old boss Boyd. Like many other up-and-coming entertainers, his career was interrupted by the war, and after serving in the Navy and seeing action in the Pacific, he reorganized his band and became a major Tulsa attraction—one big enough to have had an impact on Leon McAuliffe's postwar band. As McAuliffe noted in his 1977 *Tulsa*

Tribune interview, "I thought, well, Johnnie Lee is entrenched here and Art Davis is pretty strong and I want to be something different. So I got together a 12-piece band, a pop band..."

While Clyde Donnell "Spade" Cooley is indeed an Oklahoma native—born in 1910 near the now-defunct town of Grand—from all accounts he wasn't an Okie very long. A classically trained violinist, he ultimately landed in California, where he spent some time working with western-movie hero Roy Rogers and, later, led the West Coast's most famous western-swing outfit. And if Bob Wills' early '40s Playboys blurred the line between western-swing and contemporary swing bands, Cooley's uptown-sounding orchestra all but obliterated it. Featuring a harp and arrangements that often reflected Cooley's classical training, the group became a huge success in the 1940s, its audiences swelled by the legion of folks from the Southwest and Midwest who'd come to the West Coast to find relief from the Dust Bowl and, later, to land jobs in the defense industry. That was Bob Wills' audience, too—and, occasionally, his brother Johnnie Lee's.

O.W. Mayo remembered a show at the Santa Monica Ballroom, where Johnnie Lee and Spade squared off. "We were in California in 1947, and we played double-band dates there," he recalled. "It was the biggest ballroom I'd ever seen. Had an airplane in it. We did a battle of the bands, a double-band dance, with Johnnie Lee and the Boys and Spade and his band. He had a band pretty much like Johnnie Lee's. It was a good band."

However, it apparently wasn't good enough—or, at least, well-enough known—to go national. Said Mayo:

Spade, he made a tour, and he got back East and wasn't getting along too well. He was trying to get back to the Coast and he didn't have any dates. So he called me and wanted to know if I could sit him in.

I said, "Tell you what I'll do, Spade. I'll sit you in, and give you a percentage." I gave him a big percentage; I don't know what. And I said, "We'll plug you on the air on our show, and we'll try to get you as good a crowd as we can, but we've got the rodeo this week." [The Johnnie Lee Wills Stampede rodeo was an annual Tulsa event for decades.] So his band came in, and he came out to the rodeo and stayed until after the grand entry, then he came down here [to the Cain's Ballroom] and joined 'em, and he had a pretty good crowd. What he was trying to do was just get his band back to California.

In his *Southwest Shuffle* (Routledge, 2003), the western-swing historian and author Rich Kienzle differs with Mayo's estimation of Cooley's Cain's Ballroom crowd, calling it a "pitifully puny audience of 400." Whatever the case, Cooley managed to get back to the West Coast, where he continued to play and record, doing radio and television well past the heyday of western swing. Sadly, he may be best known these days not for his classy take on western-swing music, but for the brutal murder of his wife in 1961, for which he received a life term in prison.

Interestingly enough, the term "western swing" was apparently coined in the 1940s to help describe Cooley and his sound. (Before that, western-swing music was called a number of things: fiddle-band music, hot string-band music, and hot hillbilly music, among others.) Kienzle's *Southwest Shuffle* features a quote from western-swing bandleader, musician, and comic performer Hank Penny—who worked extensively with and around Cooley—about how Spade didn't want to be seen as simply a copy of Bob Wills.

"So what he had to do was take the idea of western swing and dress it up a la Benny Goodman, only go all with strings," said Penny, adding that "all of a sudden someone came up with the idea" of calling Cooley the King of *Western* Swing, as a play on Goodman's nickname, the King of Swing. While Penny—and author Kienzle—attribute the moniker to an unnamed source, O. W. Mayo was pretty sure he knew who came up with it.

"You always hear about King of Western Swing, king of this, king of that," said Mayo. "Roy Rogers dubbed him [Cooley] the King of Western Swing at one time—you know how a guy does. So he played that up a little bit.

"Of course," he added with a grin, "they called Bob the King of Western Swing, too."

Another man who could legitimately lay claim to that crown—he even recorded a song called "King of Western Swing"—is Hank Thompson, another Texan who settled for years in Oklahoma. Born in Waco, an octogenarian Thompson was still touring with his Brazos Valley Boys on the eve of Oklahoma's Centennial. In early 2006, he and his band opened a Tulsa date on country star Don Williams' farewell tour. Williams was seven years old when Hank recorded his debut single.

"In August, it'll be 60 years since I cut my first record, 'Whoa Sailor' with 'Swing Wide Your Gate of Love,'" he said in an interview promoting the show. "That was in August of '46 at Sellers Studios in Dallas. It was about the only recording studio in Texas then—I think there was another one in Houston. Recording equipment was very expensive. You had to cut songs on an acetate. It was quite a deal."

In the early 1950s, Hank changed his base of operations from Texas to Oklahoma City. Not long before, Bob Wills had moved his own Texas Playboys from Oklahoma City to Dallas, Texas, where he'd opened the fabulous but ill-fated dancehall called the Bob Wills Ranch

House. The two moves were not unrelated. Bob and the Playboys had been headquartered at the Oklahoma City's Trianon Ballroom, an important western-swing venue. Thompson had also played it, with promising results. He figured with Bob out of the immediate way, he could build a following by playing the Trianon. He was right.

Meanwhile, Thompson became a reliable hit-maker for Capitol Records, with his huge hit "Wild Side of Life" setting the table for dozens more charted country songs over the next several decades. In fact, Thompson is the only act to have singles on the country charts in six straight decades, from the '40s through the '90s. Along the way, he joined up with a budding music impresario named Jim Halsey, whose Tulsa-based music agency of the '70s and the '80s will be covered in a later chapter. Together, Thompson and Halsey blazed trails and set records, and while the two are no longer professionally affiliated, each continues to add to his legendary career well into the 21st Century.

While Tulsa is better known as a western-swing town, largely because of the trailblazing efforts of Bob Wills' daily KVOO broadcasts from the Cain's Ballroom—as well as brother Johnnie Lee's creditable filling of those shoes after Bob left—Oklahoma City was home to its share of notable performers as well. One of the top OKC-based acts was Merl Lindsay and His Oklahoma Nite Riders, a 1940s and '50s group that employed such well-known Oklahoma swingsters as guitarists Benny Garcia and Don Tolle, steel-guitarists Buster Magness and Gene Crownover, and saxophonist Rudy Martin. In *Saddle Serenaders* (Gibbs Smith, 1995), authors Guy Logsdon, Mary Rogers, and William Jacobson note that "many of the [Lindsay] band members moved back and forth from his band to other western swing bands, such as those led by Bob Wills, Johnnie Lee Wills, Leon McAuliffe and Hank Thompson."

Lindsay and the Nite Riders spent some time in California, but most of their work was done in Oklahoma City, where they had radio shows on several stations, including the powerhouse WKY. According to *Saddle Serenaders*, country star Red Foley appropriated Lindsay and the group in 1957 to become the house band for his TV show, "Ozark Jubilee."

Two other bandleaders with Oklahoma ties featured the state's name as a part of their own. According to Carney and Foley in *The Oklahoma Music Guide*, Illinois native Al Clauser named his band the Oklahoma Outlaws before he, or any of his bandmates, ever set foot in the state. Later, however, he and the group came to Tulsa, where they broadcast daily over radio station KTUL (the one Bob Wills had almost auditioned for back in 1934). That was in the 1940s and Clauser soon found himself competing for the same local audiences as Johnnie Lee Wills, Leon McAuliffe and Art Davis.

Even after the band's days ended, guitarist-vocalist Clauser stayed in Tulsa and made the transition to television. Locally, he may be best remembered—at least by baby boomers—as Uncle Zeke, the side-kick to Uncle Zeb on his long-running kids' show on KTUL-TV. And while he cut some fine sides, mostly for small labels, history may judge more important the early work he did with a young singer named Clara Ann Fowler, a Claremore native who, as Patti Page, would go on to become one of the bestselling female pop recording artists of all time.

Born in Pawhuska, multi-instrumentalist and singer Jimmie Revard reversed the Bob Wills path, heading to Texas and naming his band the Oklahoma Playboys. Never actually based in Oklahoma, Revard followed the pattern of radio shows, dancehall dates, and recording sessions throughout the latter half of the 1930s. Following a change of home base to Coffeyville, Kansas, the band broke up and Revard got out of the full-time bandleading business, appearing only sporadically as a performer thereafter.

Revard recorded a lot, while another act with Coffeyville ties didn't record at all. As Wilson J. "Tex" Bynum remembered in a 1990 interview, "We had thought about making records, but back at that time there was really no place you could record besides Nashville, and we just didn't get around to it."

Maybe he didn't really need to. Beginning his career in 1932 with a show on Coffeyville station KGGF, he and his Cowboys (initially the Rogers County Cowboys) found steady employment throughout the late '30s and into the early '40s, playing "dances, theaters, fairs, schools, rodeos, picnics, food stores, just anything," including dances at a long-gone Tulsa venue called the Moarra Ballroom. His reminiscences of the Moarra indicate just what a hold western swing had on Tulsa at that time.

They built this large dancehall out by Cain's—next door, really—for large traveling orchestras. The fellow who had it didn't care much for country music. But the big bands weren't doing no good when he'd book them.

One night I went out to the place and there was this 20-piece traveling orchestra up on stage and not more than eight or 10 couples in the place. I talked to the man, and he agreed to let me come out with my band. We'd play awhile, and this orchestra would play awhile. Of course, we took our own crowd with us and had a good turnout.

The man hired us, and the traveling orchestra busted up. I hired three of 'em myself, kept them in Oklahoma.

Some didn't record. Some didn't even tour much. But all of the western-swing bands that came along in the wake of Bob Wills and the Texas Playboys—whether in Oklahoma, Texas, California, or elsewhere—were working from the manual that Wills wrote. Western swing, as Bob Wills both refined and defined it from his Tulsa base, was dance music played at least partially with "hillbilly" or string-band instruments (guitars, fiddles, etc.) that featured jazz-style improvisations over the beat. Even though they were seen as corny and unsophisticated in some quarters, western swing bands had to be able to credibly handle all sorts of danceable music—even the pop hits of the day.

Truitt Cunningham, a vocalist and bassist who worked with Bob and Billy Jack Wills in the mid-'50s, tells the story of a group of tuxedo-clad swells and their dates in evening gowns who crashed a Wills dance in California one evening, striding to the front of the ballroom and sneeringly requesting Glenn Miller's big-band smash "Tuxedo Junction." According to Cunningham, Wills looked at them a moment, said, "I believe we can do that," and launched the band into a letter-perfect version of the tune, as the abashed interlopers skulked away through the crowd.

As we'll see in a few pages, the first wave of western swing lasted well into the '50s, until it was supplanted by rock 'n' roll and rockabilly music. In the 1970s, its popularity jumped up again, thanks to the efforts of hipster revivalists like Asleep at the Wheel, Commander Cody and His Lost Planet Airmen and Oklahoma City-born Alvin Crow with his Pleasant Valley Boys, along with the visibility of Bob Wills' Original Texas Playboys—the Leon McAuliffe-led group organized after Wills' death—and Texas singer-songwriter Red Steagall (whose longtime manager is Claremore's Ray Bingham) and his Coleman County Cowboys, among others. Since those days, western swing has never reached the heights it soared to during the '30s and '40s, but it's never died away again, either. These days, another Oklahoma native, the noted producer and musician Tommy Allsup, has assumed the legacy-maintaining position of Bob Wills' Original Texas Playboys—who helmed a number of Bob Wills records, including his final one, *For the Last Time*—and Texas' Leon Rausch, the Playboys' last great vocalist and lead singer for Bob Wills' Original Texas Playboys. Together, they lead outfits with former Bob and Johnnie Lee Wills sidemen—complemented, because of ever-increasing necessity, by other western swing players—in shows all around the country, including a yearly celebration of Bob Wills' March 6th birthday at the Cain's Ballroom. Other annual events celebrate Wills and his music throughout each year, including the massive get-together in Bob's old hometown of Turkey, Texas.

In 2005, the 100th anniversary of Bob's birth, Allsup and Rausch called in a number of recording acts, ranging from country superstars George Jones and Merle Haggard to R&B vocalist Archie Bell, to cut a Bob Wills tribute CD. Released on Allsup's Common Ground label, the disc includes a version of "Milk Cow Blues" sung by Cody Canada, lead vocalist and guitarist for Cross Canadian Ragweed—one of the biggest of the Oklahoma-born Red Dirt music acts (which we'll deal with in a later chapter).

"After I was done, Leon Rausch said to me, 'Well, how does it feel to be the youngest Texas Playboy?'" Canada recalled in a 2005 conversation. "I teared up."

Although he was born the year after Bob Wills died, Canada's reaction to Rausch's comment indicates that the threads of brotherhood don't just connect the Oklahoma musicians who played together, or even the bands that existed at the same time in the same places. Instead, they connect the voices and sounds, thoughts and feelings, of all the Oklahoma artists who strove, and continue to strive, to create their own kinds of music, fondly acknowledging what existed before them even as they use it and its living memory to help create something shining and new.

⮕

One of Bob's worst faults, I guess you could call it a fault, he was raised to do what he said he would do...His word was his bond. This cost him thousands, trusting people. But this was his way of life. How do you condemn a man for living by these standards? It may be bad business, but it was not bad morals. Wouldn't it be nice if everybody lived by Bob's standards?

— *Eldon Shamblin,* QUOTED IN CHARLES R. TOWNSEND'S

SAN ANTONIO ROSE

The musical legacy of Bob Wills is indisputable. More than any other single person, he was responsible for the creation and popularization of the musical genre we know as western swing. And he brought it to full fruition while living in Tulsa, Oklahoma, after planting the seed and helping the green shoot poke through the earth in his native Texas soil. Those from that proud state often call this music Texas swing (just as Red Dirt music becomes Texas music once it crosses the Red River), and while there's no doubt Texas played a major role in its creation and proliferation, that designation simply leaves out a big—arguably the *biggest*—part of the story.

But what about another important part? Are there any indications that the sense of brotherhood, community, and charity that many say typify the Oklahoma spirit lived in Wills himself?

Well, yes. In fact, there are plenty. And his longtime associate Eldon Shamblin was well qualified to comment on them. As Shamblin noted:

To many people Bob Wills had a bad reputation. They talk about his drinking and all. That's the only thing you hear; you don't hear the good things. But he had so much compassion.

There was a benefit for Bob back in 1970 [organized in Tulsa by Ruby Shamblin, Eldon's wife, to help defray Wills' medical expenses], and it was in the middle of winter with the temperature at about four degrees. We didn't think anybody'd come out, but it drew about 11,000 people. We used to say that of those 11,000 people in the audience, Bob'd probably helped half of 'em or more. That's the kind of guy he was.

One of the ways Wills helped folks was by playing funerals and insisting on never taking a dime for doing it. One of the most poignant of those funerals was for a young polio victim named Earl Edward Basse, a six-year-old who'd been a regular attendee at the Cain's Ballroom noon broadcasts, where he'd struck up a friendship with Wills. After Earl Edward's death from pneumonia, Bob and several band members, including Tommy Duncan and Joe Frank Ferguson, performed "No Disappointments in Heaven" and "Mother, Put My Little Shoes Away" for the crowd of 600 at the Sperry First Christian Church.

It happened in 1937, but Earl Edward's brother Jack Basse still recalled Wills' presence vividly in a 2006 conversation. "I remember him coming to the family car and talking to my mother and dad, big old tears coming down his face," Basse said. "It was quite a tragedy for our family, but we all appreciated what he did. And after that, it just seemed like Bob Wills was a real person."

Stories abound of Wills turning down money from promoters or dancehall owners when weather or other conditions kept crowds from coming out. As Shamblin noted in the above quote, it may not have been good business, but it was another example of what Wills felt honor-bound to do to help the people around him. The steel-guitarist Bobby Koefer, an integral part of the Wills bands in the early '50s who continues to appear with the Wills tribute bands today, recently noted how "Wills always expected his men to interact with the public and was never happy about his people being overcharged to see him and the Playboys."

We played Ruidoso, New Mexico, one time in 1951. The promoters were charging five dollars per person, which was very high in those days, Eldon told Bob about it and he had a fit. Bob said, "Why, that's terrible. That's too much for our people to have to pay, even to see [big-band leader] Harry James."

That tells you how he thought and what kind of

a person he was, even though he was twice as hot as Harry James.

In her 1937 book *Hubbin' It*, author Ruth Sheldon cited examples of Wills' generosity and compassion, including a "dying fiddler" revived after Bob came to his bedside, where he "played tune after tune for more than an hour," and an ancient fan spending her 110th birthday at the county poor farm, only to be surprised by Bob and the boys blowing in for a full-scale celebration. But she saved the most poignant example of Wills' sense of brotherhood and concern for others for the very end of the book.

Sometime in the future when the day arrives when he knows he has given all he can give he wants to say good-bye before the public has a chance to tire of him. While he is still "tops" he will give one last, glorious, farewell dance and disappear.

By that time, he plans to have bought a big ranch where the land is fertile and cheap. Scattered around the main ranch will be smaller ones for each of his boys. Without him they could not make a living elsewhere. They are too dependent upon him. He wants them always close at hand where he can take care of them and still given them orders. They will form a self-sufficient little colony with their wives and children and there will be no worries in their old age, for Bob will supervise everything, seeing that the ranch is a success just as he has made the music business a success for them.

In the evenings they will gather in the main ranch house to talk. They will bring their instruments and strike up a tune or two. They will be Bob's own Texas Playboys and when the music rises, Bob will give one of his inimitable yells of "AH-haaa" which come only when he is pleased and happy and which have brought smiles to so many thousands.

It didn't quite happen that way, but that doesn't make it any less real. And if that's not an Okie's dream, what is?

⁓

Several cats wanted me to do some arrangements for them. Out of all them great arrangers, they thought I had something special—[I had] that western swing.

—*Oklahoma City Blue Devil Buster Smith,* QUOTED IN DOUGLAS HENRY DANIEL'S *ONE O'CLOCK JUMP*

One of the staples of Bob Wills' repertoire was an instrumental called "South," which he made into a showcase fiddle tune. "South," however, was written and first performed by Bennie Moten, the Kansas City-based bandleader who hired so many of the Oklahoma City Blue Devils in the '30s. It's just one example of how Oklahoma's black and white musicians were connected as far back as the '20s and '30s. We've talked about Bob Wills' affinity for African-American blues music before; it's often been noted that his favorite singer was Bessie Smith. But trying to ascertain just how much of an influence the state's black musicians had on western swing—and, conversely, how much the white western-swing musicians had on Oklahoma's brand of jazz and blues—is tricky and probably futile. There's just no way to quantitatively measure it.

Still, it's there. The times and places might have militated against it in those segregated times, but the state's musicians could always find ways to extend their brotherhood across the then-significant barriers of color.

Pianist Clarence Cagle, a linchpin of the Johnnie Lee Wills band for many years, began playing as a teenager in his native Oklahoma City. In a 1999 interview, he remembered jamming with a young guitarist who'd have a marked influence on jazz and swing, albeit not the western kind.

We were at the Moonlight Gardens, and Charlie Christian was playing right next door in a band at the Roosevelt Inn; his brother Eddie was the leader. I'd go over on our breaks and sit behind the band-stand and listen to 'em. And every Tuesday night, I believe, we'd all meet and jam. They were jazz and we were country, but we'd play songs like "Tea for Two."

That started around 1933. In 1938, Charlie went right from our club in Oklahoma City to Benny Goodman's orchestra.

It should be noted that the clubs Cagle mentioned were in and around the Deep Deuce area of Oklahoma City, where the Oklahoma City Blue Devils had been born and flourished a decade earlier.

3
CHAPTER THREE
THIS LAND IS OUR LAND

BECAUSE of the volume and historical significance of his work, Woody Guthrie is the single most important Anglo-American folk singer of the twentieth century.
— George O. Carney and Hugh W. Foley Jr. in *Oklahoma Music Guide*

WOODY, I think, gave American music a conscience.
—John Cooper of the Red Dirt Rangers

The two most enduring music figures to emerge from the clouds of Dust Bowl-era Oklahoma, Bob Wills and Woodrow Wilson Guthrie, are both seen today as champions of the working people, artists who continually demonstrated their empathy with the economically depressed but eternally hopeful farmers and ranchers and blue-collar workers that formed the core of their audiences. It's another example of the strong spirit of brotherhood, the sense of community, that links the musicians of this state.

The connections Wills and Woody Guthrie had with their people, however, often expressed themselves in different ways, perhaps in part because of the diverse ways they'd been raised. Wills, as we've seen, had come to Tulsa from Texas, where he was no stranger to the hard labors of field and farm work. Okemah native Guthrie, while having to endure many family difficulties during his youth, came from much more of a white-collar background. As the noted music historian and performer Dr. Guy Logsdon explained it in a recent conversation, "Woody's father was the first county clerk elected in Okfuskee County in 1907, and he had land holdings. So he was what you would call a middle-class successful businessman, until family tragedies—his daughter's death in 1918, his wife's illness—bit by bit took it all away."

Interestingly, Guthrie dressed down in his public appearances, perhaps as a way of identifying with the people he cared about, while Wills and his band always dressed smartly in matching suits when they took the stage.

Then, of course, there was the music. Wills' danceable numbers offered respite from hard lives, small vacations from the challenging circumstances

> **"THE TWO MOST ENDURING MUSIC FIGURES TO EMERGE FROM THE CLOUDS OF DUST BOWL-ERA OKLAHOMA, BOB WILLS AND WOODROW WILSON GUTHRIE, ARE BOTH SEEN TODAY AS CHAMPIONS OF THE WORKING PEOPLE, ARTISTS WHO CONTINUALLY DEMONSTRATED THEIR EMPATHY WITH THE ECONOMICALLY DEPRESSED BUT ETERNALLY HOPEFUL FARMERS AND RANCHERS AND BLUE-COLLAR WORKERS THAT FORMED THE CORE OF THEIR AUDIENCES."**

of the rigors of a rural or working-class life in Depression-era America. His purpose, as he saw it, was to give those folks the best entertainment he and his bands could muster. Also, by taking requests and insisting that his musicians interact with their audiences, he made the people who listened on KVOO and attended his dances feel as though they were part of something greater—the extended Bob Wills family.

There was some of that in Woody Guthrie, too, as writer and Guthrie scholar Thomas Conner noted in recent correspondence.

Riding in boxcars and jalopies back and forth between Oklahoma and Texas and Nebraska and Colorado and California and a thousand points between them all, he found that the old folk songs, even hymns, were what people responded to. Sitting in the shadows, hungry and either too cold or too hot, suffering from the euphoria of milk-and-honey dreams or the discovery that they ditched their homes for nothing, when someone started playing the songs that reminded them of the family band back in the Woodward County living room, they brightened up and sang along and cried and slapped Woody on the back and begged for more, dear God, keep playing.

But when Guthrie began writing his own songs, they increasingly came out as something other than pure entertainment. From the mid-'30s on, Guthrie's lyrics often addressed the hardships of the people he knew, those forced off their land and onto the road as well as those still trying to eke a living in the ravaged earth of the Dust Bowl. In their *Oklahoma Music Guide*, authors George O. Carney and Hugh W. Foley Jr. note the exact date and time that Guthrie's music began dealing with the real-life situations of desperate people.

[T]he event that would shape Woody's identity as a musician and folksinger occurred on April 14, 1935. As a result of a long drought, thousands of tons of topsoil roared through the Oklahoma and Texas panhandles and covered Pampa [Texas] in a heavy dirt blanket. Following the dust were migrants, fliers in their hands that promised work in the verdant fields and valleys in California. The stories they told and the experiences of living through the dust storm and the Great Depression caused Woody to start writing the first of his dust bowl songs.

While Bob Wills occasionally recorded a song dealing at least obliquely with the conditions created by the Dust Bowl—Cindy Walker's "Dusty Skies" comes immediately to mind—or other contemporary topics, his music was meant to take his crowds' minds away from their reality and into the liberating high life of the dancehall—or, to simply help loosen a listener's heart and soul, to temporarily replace the constant drudgery in too many lives with something transcendent and captivating.

By contrast, beginning in the late '30s Woody Guthrie's songs are as often as not pleas for social change, for helping the disadvantaged, for giving the little guy a break.

Perhaps the best way to sum up the different approaches of the two men is to note the sign Guthrie famously affixed to the front of his guitar. It read, "This Machine Kills Fascists." It's nearly impossible to imagine Bob Wills slapping a sticker like that on his fiddle.

> "BORN IN OKEMAH IN 1912, WOODY GUTHRIE WAS STILL A TEENAGER WHEN HE HIT THE ROAD, NOT BOTHERING TO STAY IN SCHOOL LONG ENOUGH TO GRADUATE."

You know, Woody left the state at 17 and for all intents and purposes, never came back. Yet he was always known first and foremost as an Oklahoman. It was an inextricable and primary part of his identity. On the LA radio show, he was billed as "Oklahoma Woody." The drawl never diminished. The corn-pone humor became his stock in trade. You could look at it cynically and say he was exploiting it for a living, but he never made a living.

—*Thomas Conner*

Born in Okemah in 1912, Woody Guthrie was still a teenager when he hit the road, not bothering to stay in school long enough to graduate. His family had pretty much gone to pieces by that time anyway. As Guy Logsdon noted earlier, Woody's sister had died when he was six—in a gruesome ironing accident involving kerosene—and Woody's mother had been taken off to Central State Hospital in Norman because of Huntington's disease, which at that time was wrongly considered a mental condition. His father was away from home as well, at least partly because of Woody's mother's affliction.

"Huntington's disease involves a great deal of involuntary movement, of jerking," explained Logsdon. "If she had a cup of coffee in her hand, she might jerk it, and it would splash on someone, and people would say, 'Oh, she's mad. She's crazy.' It was that involuntary movement that caused her husband's burns."

So Woody's mother went to an institution, his father relocated to Pampa, Texas—where he had sisters to help him recover from his burns—and Woody was left alone in Okemah. There, noted Logsdon, "he stayed mostly by himself for two years."

Eventually, Woody joined his dad in Pampa, got married, and started performing in a hillbilly-style band called the Corncob Trio. After the 1935 epiphany described earlier, he hit the road, ending up in California—where, for a time, he hosted a radio show with his singer/construction worker cousin Jack Guthrie, who would have a major World War II-era hit with one of Woody's most famous compositions, the richly nostalgic "Oklahoma Hills."

Like California author John Steinbeck, whose first-hand witness of the brutal conditions facing American migrant workers in his home state led to the classic novel *Grapes of Wrath*, Guthrie's experience with the homeless and dispossessed—many of whom came from the same area of the country as he did—politicized his music even more. He became a champion of labor unions and a voice for the working classes who during the Great Depression must've often felt as though they had no public voice at all.

Because of his identification with the blue-collar working people, and the polemic content of many of his songs, Guthrie became identified with the workers'-rights movements of the 1930s. In the minds of some—most of them *not* members of the working classes—it was at this point that Woody Guthrie became a communist. Certainly, there's no denying that he played for communist-related events and that his music advocated the sharing of wealth with the poor rather than unfettered profit-above-everything capitalism. But, as Logsdon noted, it wasn't quite that simple.

Woody wasn't a card-carrying Commie. He wasn't a card-carrying *anything*.

Jim Longhi wrote a book called Woody, Cisco and Me *[University of Illinois Press, 1997], and many years ago in New York he told me the story of one night when he and Woody and Cisco Houston were in the bottom of a Merchant Marine ship during World War II. They're talking, and Woody says, "Sometimes they said my mother was insane. I don't think she was. But sometimes I think I've got the same disease that she had—and if I do, only Jesus Christ can save me."*

Jim said, "Woody, I didn't know you were religious."

He said, "Oh, yeah, I like 'em all. I just don't have a favorite."

"He also said that his favorite two people in history were Jesus Christ and Will Rogers," added Logsdon. "Those are not the words of a dirty commie pinko."

"HE ALSO SAID THAT HIS FAVORITE TWO PEOPLE IN HISTORY WERE JESUS CHRIST AND WILL ROGERS," ADDED LOGSDON. "THOSE ARE NOT THE WORDS OF A DIRTY COMMIE PINKO."

"To me, what he did was just a plain-spoken everyman-ness," said John Cooper of the Oklahoma-based band the Red Dirt Rangers in a recent interview. "He sang about the search for truth and justice, about every person's right to that truth and justice. He gave people who didn't have a voice a voice, and he spoke it eloquently. He was the voice of the displaced Okies."

In 1940, Guthrie left the West Coast, traveling across the country and landing in New York, where he continued to champion unions and workers' rights. It was during this time that he composed his best-known song, "This Land Is Your Land." And while the classic tune can be seen as an upbeat celebration of America's wonderful diversity and how lucky we all are to live in the greatest country in the world, it's also got plenty of bite. As Thomas Conner has pointed out, Guthrie conceived it as a protest song, written in heated response to Irving Berlin's "God Bless America."

"Woody saw that kind of passivity as inherently dangerous," wrote Conner of Guthrie's quarrel with the sentiments in "God Bless America." "That's why so many friends and family had lost their farms. If they'd only come together and stood their ground, so to speak, things might have been different. He wanted people to realize what was theirs. This land—it's yours. This music—it's yours.

"What constituted ownership to Woody?" he added. "Work. You worked this land, you have a stake in it. That's your blood in it."

Guthrie didn't just preach those ideas. He lived them as well.

"His early royalty structure was pretty screwed up," noted Conner, "because he just didn't see how he could own something like a song."

Logsdon agreed. "Woody wrote new lyrics, but he used old melodies that he just modified a little bit. And he had a philosophy: 'These songs didn't cost me anything, so you can have 'em if you want 'em.'"

In the '40s, Guthrie recorded for the famed folk-music scholar Alan Lomax as well as for major-label RCA, which first released a number of his songs under the collective title of *Dust Bowl Ballads*. He also performed in the Almanac Singers, a group that would later, without Guthrie, become the Weavers, a folk group that saw considerable mainstream success in post World War II America, (especially with the old folk ballad "Goodnight, Irene," which became a multimillion seller for the group in the early 1950s).

After his wartime service in the Merchant Marine, Guthrie returned to New York and

> "WOODY WROTE NEW LYRICS, BUT HE USED OLD MELODIES THAT HE JUST MODIFIED A LITTLE BIT. AND HE HAD A PHILOSOPHY: 'THESE SONGS DIDN'T COST ME ANYTHING, SO YOU CAN HAVE 'EM IF YOU WANT 'EM.'"

continued to play and record. Sadly, the comments he'd made to his shipmates Jim Longhi and Cisco Houston came true, and he began experiencing the oncoming symptoms of Huntington's disease, the same physiological malady that had stricken his mother. By the early 1950s, he was no longer able to perform, and he spent the last 13 years of his life in a series of hospitals, as the degenerative muscle disease slowly leached its irreversible toll. Before his 1967 death, he was visited by many artists who were becoming a part of the revitalized folk-music movement of the 1960s, including its leading light, Bob Dylan.

"If Woody Guthrie had only inspired one artist, Bob Dylan—which he did—he would've changed music forever," said John Cooper. "But he did so much more. Some say he was the first noted American singer-songwriter. Of course, you can go all the way back to Stephen Foster and make a case there. But you'd have to say that Woody Guthrie was the first singer-songwriter with a social conscience."

Woody's probably ten times more famous now than when he was alive, both here and overseas. It goes back to Dylan, and even to the Weavers, if you want to go back that far. Worldwide, he may be the most famous Oklahoman.

— *John Cooper*

As George O. Carney and Hugh W. Foley Jr. point out in their *Oklahoma Music Guide*, Woody Guthrie lived to see the '60s folk revival that bore his distinct influence. He was, however, unable to participate in it. By the time of his death in 1967, he'd long been unable to play, sing, or write.

He was, however, there in spirit, and while that's surely a cliché, it has a much deeper meaning in Guthrie's case. His influence on the whole '60s movement, which encompassed artists like Dylan, former Oklahomans Tom Paxton and Duncan native Hoyt Axton, and even Guthrie's own son, Arlo—among many others—was distinctly spiritual. Much of the folk music that emerged from that era continued in the Guthrie spirit of reaching out and bringing people together and then, once you had them listening, illuminating social injustices.

That leads to the question of how much Guthrie, and by extension, the folk music that followed him, had to do with Oklahoma. In a recent work called *"Getting Along: Woody Guthrie and Oklahoma's Red Dirt Musicians,"* slated for publication in 2007, Thomas Conner quoted Guthrie's daughter Nora, who spoke to him just before the 2002 opening of a traveling Smithsonian exhibit of Guthrie memorabilia.

Everything he did and fought for had to do with the basic values he learned in Oklahoma. When I lecture in Oklahoma, I tell people, "You think he's

talking about other people's rights and other people's problems, but he was talking about your grandfather"—and I point at them—"and your aunt and your cousin. These were his people. Everything he wrote, especially the early songs, was about your family."... Everything he cared about came from his love for Oklahoma and then became explained and justified by the rest of his life...

Oklahoma has reciprocated with some love of its own, although there are still those in the state—including in Guthrie's home town—who haven't been willing or able to reconcile themselves with his alleged commie leanings. As Logsdon has pointed out, this linkage of Guthrie and the communists reached its peak during the Red Scare years of the 1950s, when Senator Joseph McCarthy "came out and convinced everyone that if you had a social conscience, you were a communist." But old accusations and prejudices die hard, and it took a while for the state to really embrace one of its most influential native sons.

Conner marks 1988 as the year when the anti-Guthrie sentiment began waning in his hometown and home state. That year, Minnesota folksinger Larry Long, working in the Okemah schools as an artist in residence, gave a concert that drew attention to Guthrie and his work. He came back to Okemah for a similar show the next year, and the year after, Arlo Guthrie played in Okemah—his first concert in his dad's hometown.

It took a few more years, but in 1998, the first annual Woody Guthrie Free Folk Festival was held during a hot Okemah summer, bringing in musicians and fans from all across the country and beyond. In 1997, the year before the inaugural Guthrie festival, the Muskogee-based, newly formed Oklahoma Music Hall of Fame included Woody in its first group of inductees.

Guthrie's legacy, of course, extends well beyond his Dust Bowl ballads and workers'-rights songs of the '30s and '40s, and the long shadow he cast over the folk-music revival of the 1960s. As we'll see in a later chapter, his populist spirit of brotherhood and social conscience also infuses the work of Oklahoma's Red Dirt musicians, a group of singer-songwriters working in a variety of musical styles but all inspired

> **"ASCERTAINING WHAT WOODY DID THAT WAS GENUINELY DIFFERENT IS NOT EASY. HE REALLY DIDN'T DO MUCH THAT WAS DIFFERENT OR UNIQUE. NOT MUSICALLY. I GUESS WHAT HE DID THAT WAS DIFFERENT WAS, IN EVERY SITUATION, SIMPLY INSISTING THAT THESE SONGS, THIS MUSIC, WAS AS IMPORTANT AS ANYTHING ELSE."**

by the same common-folk concerns and sense of community and brotherhood that Woody espoused in his own songs. Like Guthrie's songs, the music of the Red Dirt movement can be hard to pin down in exact terms, until you consider that attitude and spirit are as crucial as the music itself.

As Thomas Conner wrote, "Ascertaining what Woody did that was genuinely different is not easy. He really didn't do much that was different or unique. Not musically. I guess what he did that was different was, in every situation, simply insisting that these songs, this music, was as important as anything else."

Red Dirt musician Cooper agreed. "With Woody," he said, "it wasn't the melody, it was the message, and his body of work is as relevant now, if not more relevant, than it was then. What he said is so important, man. It's so important. And we really need it now."

4
CHAPTER FOUR
TULSA FINDS A NEW SOUND

ROCK and Roll? Why, man, that's the same kind of music we've been playin' since 1928!
 —Bob Wills, quoted by Jim Downing in the January 4, 1958, *Tulsa Tribune*

BOB Wills left Cain's due to very poor crowds. This probably was caused by the rise in popularity of rock 'n' roll and country music. Swing was not selling at the time.
 —Benny Ketchum, leader of the Cain's Ballroom house band in the late '50s

Listen to Bob Wills' recordings of the early and mid-'50s, and you'll hear some music that sounds a great deal like early rock 'n' roll. Tunes like "Bottle Baby Boogie" and "(Me and My Baby) Doin' the Bunny Hop" represent attempts by the western-swing founder to keep up with the times, something he'd been doing with a decent amount of success for years.

By the late '50s, however, the times were a-changin' just a little too quickly for even a canny showman and master entertainer like Wills. Western-swing music, a powerful force in the Southwest and elsewhere for more than two decades, was in eclipse. A new generation, hungry for something fresh, was on the way up. The earliest members of a huge group of American kids born after World War II, who would come to be known collectively as baby boomers, were climbing toward adolescence. Meanwhile in a Memphis studio, a Southern boy a few years older than those boomers and some of his cohorts, whipped up a bit of alchemy that would forever change the direction of pop music. In the same way that Wills had mixed musical elements to create a new sound two decades earlier, Elvis Presley would become known as the artist who first synthesized country music and black rhythm & blues into something called rockabilly—which would later be pulled under the big tent of rock 'n' roll.

Of course, that wasn't the first time that country—then called hillbilly—music and black blues had been squeezed together to make something new. In an April 10, 2003, article in the online publication *Tulsa Today*, veteran musician and writer James McMaster Downing remembered his father, the *Tulsa Tribune's* Jim Downing, calling Bob Wills one day in 1956 and saying, "Bob, I hear a lot of talk about this Elvis Presley kid. They say the reason for his success is that he's blending White Hillbilly music with Negro Blues. Isn't that what you did?"

According to the younger Downing's story, Wills laughed and replied, "That's exactly what we were doing! We just didn't call it Rock and Roll back then."

Certainly, there were differences between what Wills and Presley did with those two components. But it's also worth noting that one of the ingredients of the revved-up new rock 'n' roll sound was western swing. Presley, after all, did a version of the Wills standard "Milk Cow Blues" in his Sun Records sessions of '55, although it was taken at a gallop instead of a lope and released in 1955 as "Milkcow Blues Boogie." Another famous early rocker, Bill Haley, led a country band that included western swing in its repertoire. Then he changed his sound and dropped down into slap-bass four-beat rockabilly mode for "Rock Around the Clock," the pioneering rock 'n' roll tune that became the first of his long string of '50s hits.

In some ways, it wasn't much of a drop from western swing to rock 'n' roll. Being first and foremost dance bands, the groups led by Bob and Johnnie Lee Wills played songs in all sorts of rhythms, from waltzes to prototypical 4/4 beat rock 'n' roll. (Johnnie Lee's group, in fact, would go on to have a Top 40 regional rock 'n' roll hit in the early '60s with "Blub's Twist," a song made up on the spot at one of the band's dances by saxophonist Glenn "Blub" Rhees.) But in other ways, there was a world of difference—primarily because the new generation, like those before them, didn't think it was particularly hip to dance to their parents' music.

By late 1957, with rockabilly and rock 'n' roll firmly established as the new American sounds, Bob Wills returned to Tulsa and the Cain's Ballroom, where Johnnie Lee was still doing the daily regional broadcasts for General Mills. Luke was also in Tulsa at the time, no longer a bandleader, playing bass with Johnnie Lee and All His Boys.

An in-depth 1958 newspaper story—a small portion of which is quoted at the beginning of this chapter—deals with Bob, Johnnie Lee, Luke and O.W. Mayo (who by then owned the Cain's), revealing a great deal about western swing's somewhat bewildered relationship with the new young music that was supplanting it. In the piece, the *Tulsa Tribune's* Jim Downing wrote that Bob and his brothers "hope to woo a third generation of youngsters away from their TV sets and record players and bring them out for dances."

In a quote later in the story, however, Bob seemed to let slip a little of how he really felt about the dominant pop music of the day. "We just keep the beat clean and hard and don't clonk it up like this so-called rock 'n' roll," he said. "If they can't dance to our rhythm, then they just plain can't dance. Period."

The problem, of course, was that the people dancing to Wills' music at the Cain's Ballroom weren't primarily kids and a good portion of his late-'50s audiences hadn't been kids for quite a long time. Nonetheless, combining players from both the Texas Playboys and Johnnie Lee's group—including Luke and Johnnie Lee himself—Bob formed a new Playboys band that played the daily broadcasts for more than two years. In 1959, however, he got a lucrative offer to headline in a Las Vegas casino, and he left for Nevada, followed by Johnnie Lee, bringing to a close the noonday KVOO broadcasts that had been a part of Oklahoma's popular culture for nearly a quarter of a century.

Bob Wills was a bright man, one who could always calculate what an audience wanted, so maybe his decision to take the Vegas gigs had to do with something more than money. After all, the audiences at the Showboat (where he went after leaving Tulsa) and, later, the Golden Nugget, were grownups, and as such would be less likely to have succumbed to the lure of rock 'n' roll.

Meanwhile, however, a new band took over at the Cain's. And while little has been written about this group, Benny Ketchum and the Western Playboys amount to more than a footnote in the history of Oklahoma music—if only because of what they represent. Ketchum, born on a farm outside of Dewey, led a group that stands, a half-century later, as the bridge between western swing and a rock 'n' roll style that would come to be known as the Tulsa Sound.

"Swing was dying, and rock 'n' roll was coming on," recalled Ketchum in a 2005 interview. "The people that were coming to Cain's were pretty well established, but you were limited. They were people that had been coming there forever.

"Well, we didn't want to lose those people. So we played enough stuff that they liked to keep 'em. Then we played enough rock 'n' roll that we drew *new* people into it."

According to Ketchum, Johnnie Lee Wills hadn't yet joined brother Bob in Las Vegas when Ketchum brought his seven-member Western Playboys to the Cain's to begin playing regular dances. He'd first grabbed the attention of Cain's manager Alvin Perry a year or so earlier, when he'd swung through on a tour with singer Bobby Helms. Helms, of "Fraulein" and "My Special Angel" fame, had a foot in both country and rock 'n' roll music, and Perry thought that might be just what the ballroom needed. Ketchum recalled, "As we went on the tour, we wound up in California, and Alvin Perry called me on the phone and said, 'You know, you guys could be the house band here if you want this.'"

It sounded good to Ketchum, who'd grown up, like so many other northeastern Oklahoma kids, listening to the Wills radio broadcasts from the Cain's. So he signed on with Perry and began playing Friday and Saturday night dances, often bringing in country and rockabilly recording artists, like Carl Perkins, to perform with the group on weekends, when the Cain's competed for attendance with Leon McAuliffe's Cimarron Ballroom.

Johnnie Lee Wills, meanwhile, "was still there, but dyin', you know, as far as crowds were concerned," remembered Ketchum. "Bob had already died. He'd gone.

"They [the Johnnie Lee Wills group] still worked the Wednesday night dances, as I recall," he added. "And then finally that disappeared, and we did Wednesday, Friday and Saturday nights.

Wednesday night was the regular dance they'd always had, so we cut back on our rock 'n' roll then and did western swing and waltzes."

The band Bob and Johnnie Lee put together when Bob returned to the Cain's was a versatile one, boasting three fiddles and three saxophones. Ketchum's smaller outfit maintained that versatility by carrying two fiddlers who also doubled as saxophonists, as well as a steel-guitarist who could also play electric guitar. The group, he said, was primarily a country act, but circumstances at the Cain's called for expertise in other types of music as well.

It was known for [western] swing, so that era we were in there became kind of a stepchild. Rock 'n' roll was big, but the people was still hanging onto western swing and country music. There's a separation there. People talk about western swing and country music. They're two different things. We came there playing country music. We used country stars. So, that just kind of mixed up until there was nothing where you could say, 'Well, this was swing, this was country, this was rock 'n' roll.' They were just fused.

Although that kind of fusion was present in a lot of the acts playing in Tulsa clubs during those days, there wasn't quite as much of a country or swing influence with the young rock 'n' rollers Ketchum knew. He was, however, always welcome in their circles.

Jimmy Markham, Leon Russell—Russell Bridges at the time—David Gates and those people were playing at the Paradise Club then. They were just kids, and I was a young man. I was 20. We had rhinestone suits, we were making money, and I'd take the stars out there with me. Boy, they just ate that up, that these big stars were there to see 'em. And we'd sit in and play rock 'n'

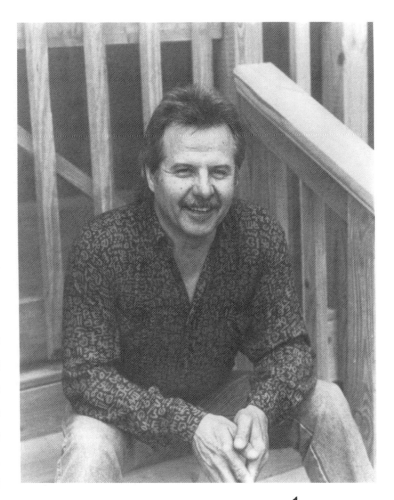

Jimmy Markham

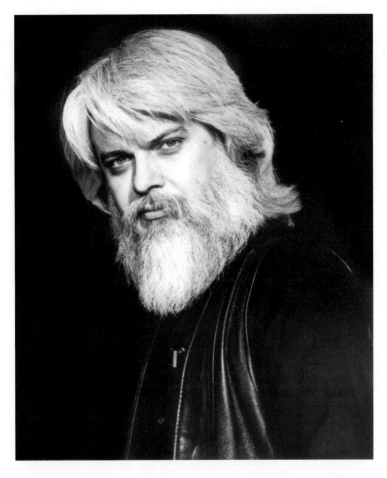

Leon Russell

country star Ernest Tubb's famous guitarist.

"He said, 'Hey, you Fabian reject—let's see if you can play some of this Billy Byrd music,'" remembered Ketchum with a laugh.

The object of Dickens' derision was a man Ketchum had plucked out of the Tulsa clubs to play with his band, a guitarist who, the bandleader noted, "was a good guitar player, but I don't think his heart was ever in country music."

Indeed, "Fabian reject" Johnny Cale wouldn't make his mark in country music. But he'd go on to a more lasting fame than the late-'50s rock 'n' roll idol Dickens compared him to—and, as J.J. Cale, would also become one of the major architects of the rock music style known as the Tulsa Sound.

roll and get free drinks and what have you.

While Ketchum and most of his out-of-town headliners mixed easily with Tulsa's rockers, some of the old-line Nashville stars he invited to headline with his band at the Cain's weren't nearly as sanguine about the practitioners of this new music. Ketchum recalled headliner Little Jimmy Dickens looking at the Western Playboys' ducktailed guitarist with disdain and invoking the name of

Oklahoma was a dry state back when we all started. Since there wasn't supposed to be any liquor, there weren't any liquor laws, and so there were a lot of clubs, a lot of places, where people could go and drink 24 hours a day. The police didn't pay any attention and there weren't any kind of rules. And since there weren't any rules, you could do anything you wanted to. It was kind of a wide-open town. When something like that happens, when people don't get caught up in that political morality, it creates kind of a hotbed of musical experience.

—*Tulsa Sound architect Leon Russell*

Russell's home state didn't repeal prohibition

until 1959, but that didn't mean for a moment that people weren't going out and drinking. To paraphrase native son Will Rogers, Oklahomans would vote against liquor as long as they could stagger to the polls.

Rogers' oft-quoted observation fits hand-in-glove with a recent comment from historian Guy Logsdon. "Oklahomans," Logsdon said, "loved to dance all Saturday night and pray all Sunday morning, and if people don't understand that, they don't understand Oklahoma. We're very religious, but we like to sin a little, too."

In late-'50s Tulsa, the sinning often came with live background music, in technically illegal nightclubs. Many of those clubs lay in the Greenwood Avenue area of north Tulsa, a place that was once such an economic force it was known as the Black Wall Street. Then came the infamous 1921 Tulsa race riots, and the whole area was destroyed, only to emerge again and eventually achieve a new reputation as a place to see and hear live music at just about any hour of the day, any time of the year. (Blues and jazz festivals and other events still unfold regularly in and around Greenwood, mostly in the summer.)

In those segregated days, the Greenwood clubs featured black music aimed toward black audiences. But a new group of young white kids, their heads and hearts opened up to blues and R&B by a pioneering Tulsa deejay named Frank Berry, began sneaking across town to hear some of that stuff played live. And before too long, some of them were playing there as well.

"Most all of the bands were blues-based over there [around Greenwood]," remembered Leon Russell in a 1999 interview. "We'd go to the shows over at the Dreamland, the Big 10 Ballroom, to see all these kinds of music-hall acts that came through there. Those places went seven nights a week, and they'd have national acts, national bands, in there. They'd have two or three acts a night. It was quite a place to see shows."

It wasn't long before he was playing piano and singing in those sorts of places himself, sometimes playing two different jobs a night. "I started working in clubs when I was 14, and, as I said, the police didn't pay any attention and there weren't any kind of rules, which suited me fine. It gave me kind of an early start."

Those early blues and R&B influences would not only have a profound effect on Leon Russell's later music, but on the style known as the Tulsa Sound as well. So would country music, even though Russell said he never played any of it during his formative musical years in Tulsa clubs.

Other seminal Tulsa rockers, however, did. In the mid-'50s, Gene Crose was enrolled at Oklahoma Military Academy in Claremore,

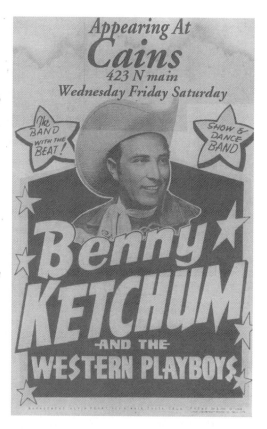

Benny Ketchum and the Western Playboys concert poster

preparing a few country songs to sing for the school's annual talent show. Then, a fellow cadet turned him onto a yellow-label 45 rpm record he'd picked up after hearing its artist, Elvis Presley, play in a theater in Odessa, Texas.

"When I heard that, country just blew out the window," recalled Crose in a 2003 interview. "It was Elvis from then on."

Although national fame eluded Crose, he was a popular Tulsa rock 'n' roller for years, and many—if not most—of the musicians who'd go on to create the Tulsa Sound played in his bands at one time or another. One of the first was Johnny Cale, only a couple of years before he joined Benny Ketchum and the Western Playboys. Remembered Crose:

I had seen Johnny with a little group called the Country Cousins. So I went over to Cale's house and literally talked him into playing for me. He said, "No, man, I can't do it. I'm not good enough." And I said, "I've heard you. I know you can do it, Johnny."

When we started playing shows, he knew one riff. That's all he could play. I had to get him with records and let him hear different things, and when he'd hit a different note I'd say, "No, it goes such and such." Now, I'm not a guitar player, but I could hear it. So that's really how he learned, just from hard work and practicing and learning the hard way.

In a 2004 conversation, Cale noted that the Country Cousins—a trio consisting of local boys Earl Dean Dobbins and Billy Mecom—did "Homer & Jethro kind of stuff," referring to the then-popular country-music parody act.

That was the first thing I did. I didn't sing or anything. Those two guys sang and I played rhythm guitar for 'em. I was still in school, and I know we would get out of school at three o'clock and get in somebody's car and play, like, Okmulgee and Sapulpa and the small towns around there. We played theater things—around the movie, you know. It was very much country.

Although he played exclusively country music then, he wasn't particularly a fan of the genre. As he explained, growing up in Tulsa in the '50s, "that's mainly what you heard."

"Of course, Bob Wills was on the radio, and the older folks all listened to Leon McAuliffe, Bob Wills, and Johnnie Lee, right? It was on the radio at noon every day on KVOO," Cale said. "And you know, I don't think I liked it or disliked it. It was just what you *heard*. The thing that really raised my attention span," he added, "was when rock 'n' roll started coming in."

Billy Mecom and Gene Crose were friends, which is how Cale came to play with Crose, crossing over from country to rock 'n' roll. Meanwhile, other hepcat singers were popping up in Tulsa and the surrounding area, organizing bands and hustling jobs. In the period between 1956, when Crose put together his first Tulsa group, and 1959, the scene exploded, producing frontmen like Clyde Stacy (who'd have a national hit in 1957 with "So Young"), Bobby Taylor, Wally Wiggins, Bill Pair, Coffeyville, Kansas-based Rodney Lay (who'd become the longtime leader of Tulsa-based country superstar Roy Clark's band), Jumpin' Jack Dunham, Jimmy Markham and Tommy Rush.

Perhaps the most unlikely of these bandleaders was a classically trained high school pianist, violinist and ukulele player. Like Russell and many of the others, he loved deejay Frank Berry's rhythm and blues show. And, Russell himself—when he was still going by his given name of Russell Bridges—played in the man's first band. But from the beginning, David Gates was a little different kind of guy. As his first bass player, Gerald Goodwin, remembered in a 2003 conversation, "He took himself seriously. He took his music seriously. He was ambitious. In the beginning, I think the rest of us were just in it for a good time."

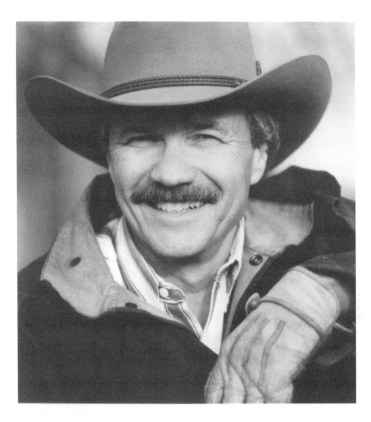

David Gates

I didn't need to do the clubs, because the parties were abundant. Clubs only paid ten dollars a night, and I could make more doing the parties than I could grinding out five hours at the clubs. You did that only when you had to.

—David Gates

I kind of moved into clubs, because I didn't have a day job. So I needed some money. I was always looking for more than a Friday and Saturday night gig.

—J.J. Cale

I was mostly a club guy. I got a little bit of an education playing those joints, I guess you'd call 'em. I remember them being packed. People packed into a booth, and the women would be carrying on. Ah. Smoke. Fights.

—DRUMMER *Chuck Blackwell*

Before rock 'n' roll came along, a young Tulsa musician didn't have many chances to play for a real audience. Tommy Crook, once cited by Chet Atkins on *The Tonight Show* for his prowess on the guitar, was one of those musicians. In 2003, he remembered playing mid-'50s country shows on movie-theater stages—just as Johnny Cale had done—with "15 or 20 different acts."

They'd have bales of hay up there—it was just like the Grand Ole Opry. A guy'd come out and introduce the acts, and most everybody had comedy. I'd tell jokes and sing those old novelty tunes, like "Smoke That Cigarette." That's how I met Cale. That's how I got started, and there wasn't anybody else doing anything then. 'Course, there wasn't any place for them to do it anyway. Back in those days, there was one all-night grocery store, the Trenton Market. And as far as restaurants and clubs, there wasn't any such thing. They didn't even really have those brown-bag things in those days, because until '59, everything was bootleg whiskey.

Before the repeal of prohibition in 1959, the only alcoholic drink that could legally be served in Oklahoma bars was beer with an alcohol content of no more than 3.2 percent. But, as Leon Russell noted earlier, there were plenty of places that didn't play by those rules, choosing instead to run the risk of the occasional bust. (The "brown-bag" clubs Crook referred to came along after '59, when it became legal to drink liquor or wine in a bar, provided that the customer bought it at a package store and brought it into the club.)

As we've seen earlier, the nightspots required live entertainment, and the young musicians inspired by rock 'n' roll found lots of work as a result. But as the music swept through teenage America, other venues opened for the new bands and their bandleaders, places where the teen musicians could legally play for people their own age. In Tulsa, high school social clubs sponsored dances, radio stations presented sock hops in gymnasiums and other kid-friendly places, and some of the dancehalls, like Leon McAuliffe's Cimarron Ballroom, started running teen nights, where soda pop replaced anything stronger, at least for the evening.

In Tulsa, many of those Tulsa Sound pioneers played both kinds of engagements—although some, like David Gates and his Accents, specialized in the teen gigs, while others—like Cale, saxophonist Johnny Williams, and bandleaders Dunham and Markham, found steady employment playing for the denizens of Tulsa's adult nightspots.

"Those guys were doing clubs and I was pretty much doing all the Central and Rogers [high school] dances and parties," noted Gates in a 2003 conversation. "There were occasional times when the other bands would do some of those, too. But we pretty much had a lock on that, because we were playing this broad spectrum of rock 'n' roll and ballads and stuff that people seemed to want. We had something for everybody."

Gates called the clubs "unrewarding—there might be people there, there might not."

On the other hand, drummer Chuck Blackwell, in a 2003 conversation, took a fonder view of playing the '50s nightspots.

I wouldn't trade what I've been through for a college education. It was too much fun. You had the orneriness. You had the ladies, the music. What else would a young man want to do but be where the party is, the good times, and be able to contribute to that? And to see people dancing to your music. Oh, I loved to watch people dance.

I had a house up in the Hollywood Hills, and I think I had 123 live-in houseguests in one year. I figured it out one day. It was kind of an active location. The neighbors, I found out in later years, thought there was a motorcycle gang that lived there, because they heard music all the time. Of course, that was the studio.

—Leon Russell

When Woody Guthrie and Bob Wills made their trips to the West Coast in the '30s and '40s, they found all sorts of homefolks there, relocated because of Great Depression-related economics and other forces, but still partial to the music they'd heard back in Oklahoma. In the '60s, another wave of Okies hit California. Like their brethren of a generation earlier, they came for the jobs—but the jobs they came for were musical.

Lore has it that Leon Russell was the first of the Tulsa Sound crowd to migrate to L.A., where he became a major session musician as well as a magnet for many of his old rock 'n' roll compadres back home. That, however, is only partially true. There were others before Leon. Apparently, the first guy from the Tulsa scene to try his luck on

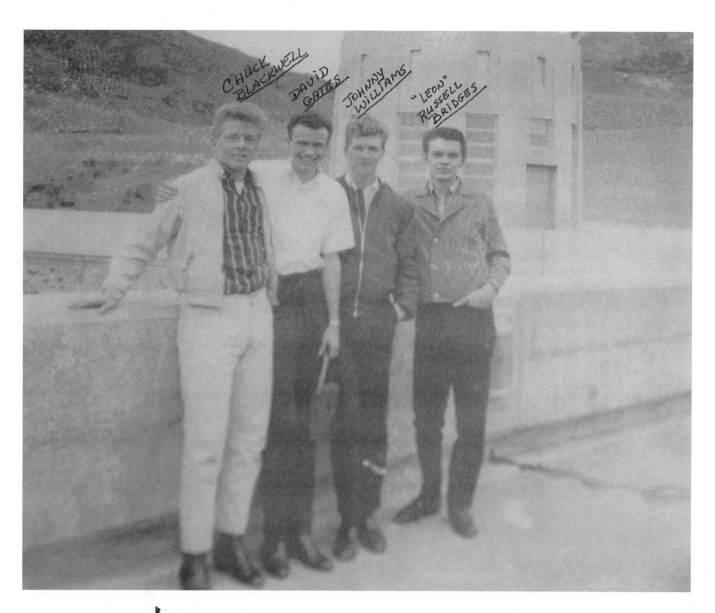

**Chuck Blackwell
David Gates
Johnny Williams
"Leon" Russell Bridges
late 1950s**

the coast was singer-guitarist Bill Pair, who left town after graduating from Will Rogers High School, taking the members of his group, the Wild Childs, along. Pair recalled his decision, and its results, in a 2004 interview.

I just thought, "What the heck? I'm this age and I'm gonna go find out what's out there." We decided we all had to have 300 dollars apiece in cash before we went to L.A. That'd give us enough to kind of hang loose until we got things going.

Then, when we got there, we thought, "Well, we've got a little bit of money..." Back then, you could do a lot of things with 300 dollars. So we'd just go to the beach and everything like that instead of looking for a job. We did get us an apartment. But then we got down to 50 cents, and I said, "Hey, now. C'm'on, guys." And I got us a gig the first place we went to.

The group settled in at a club called the Golden Arms in Torrance, and not long afterward saxophonist Johnny Williams arrived to join the band, now called Bill Pair and the Outsiders.

"I think Johnny Williams kind of spread the word," said Pair with a laugh. "Our style went over real good out there—basically, that Tulsa Sound."

We didn't have any problem drawing crowds. Then people [from Tulsa] started trickling in. Johnny was the first one. [Drummer] Jimmy Karstein came out. Chuck Blackwell. Leon [Russell]. Leon and I got us a little duo gig at a beer bar. We both needed the money, I guess. Lee Weir, a guitar player. I think he and Jack Dunham came out together.

Pair had gotten the Golden Arms gig in the summer of '59. By 1961, he was on the road, playing with B. Bumble and the Stingers, the road version of a studio band that had scored a big instrumental hit with "Bumble Boogie" that same year.

Meanwhile, the Tulsa boys kept burning up the road to California. By the early '60s, they were all over the place, playing in clubs and beginning to find their way around the L.A. studio scene. David Gates had arrived earlier, planning to bring his band, the Accents, with him.

"I had what I thought was the finest band in the world at the time, which was Carl Radle on bass, Tommy Crook on guitar, and Jimmy Karstein on drums," said Gates. "I played piano and some rhythm guitar. I *loved* playing with those guys. I got Karstein to go with me on an exploratory trip, and I begged Tommy to come. He would not come. And Carl said, 'No, no, I don't want to do it.' So I had to abandon my four-piece band."

Gates and Karstein went anyway, looking up one of the few Tulsans on the coast at the time, Jumpin' Jack Dunham, who'd made the trip in spring of 1960.

"The next two that came were Jimmy Karstein and David Gates," remembered Dunham in 2003, "and they stayed with me and my wife at the time for a week and a half, two weeks, until they found themselves jobs and a place to live."

Karstein would last about six months before heading back home, deciding to get a straight job. But the lure of the music eventually drew him back again. He'd go on to become a major West Coast studio player and a member (with Carl

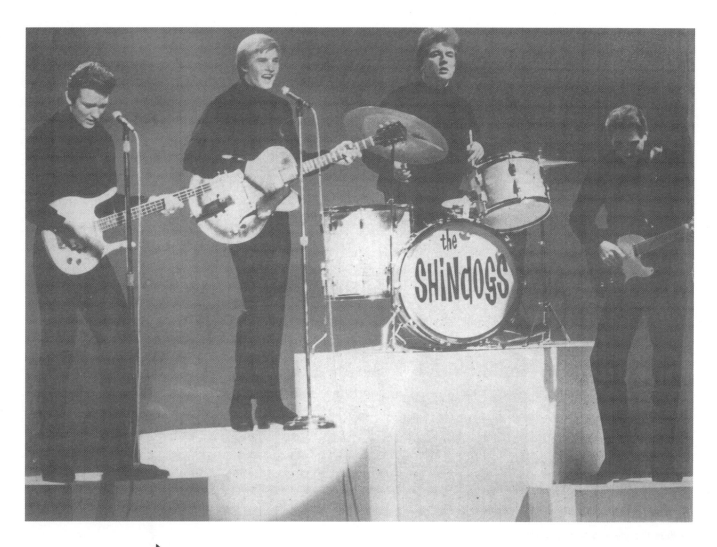

**The Shindogs
Chuck Blackwell at top**

Radle and Tulsa guitarist Tommy Tripplehorn) of '60s hitmakers Gary Lewis and the Playboys. At this writing, he lives in Tulsa, where he continues to perform with the Red Dirt Rangers and several other Oklahoma acts.

"I decided I'd made the wrong career move," Karstein said in a 2003 interview. "See, my granddad was a groceryman here in town and I thought, 'Yeah, I'd better get out of this music and go to work for him.'

A career [in music]? Nobody thought about that. You just couldn't get enough, so you went and did it. We didn't think in terms of career—well, David Gates did. But he also was five or six years older than every-

body else, and he had a family, and he'd been to New York and he'd kind of figured a few things out.

"I got Leon Russell and Chuck Blackwell to come out to California and work as a trio in clubs, while we were trying to work our way into the recording industry as studio musicians," said Gates, whose days of high school hops and social-club gigs lay behind him in Tulsa.

Chuck and Leon lived with me in Downey for eight or nine months, and then in Hollywood for almost a year. We were in Downey for a year, and Chuck and Leon were there probably the last eight or nine months of that year. I was on my own to start, and then when they came, we could work clubs together, and did so. Then I rented a house in Hollywood, and it had two floors. Chuck and Leon stayed downstairs, and ultimately Carl Radle moved in and took another bedroom, and [wife] Jo Rita and I and the two kids were upstairs.

Although Gates apparently navigated the Southern California club scene with few problems, others had a tougher time. When Russell first hit the area, for instance, he found that the nightspots in L.A. were far more regulated than the semi-legal joints back home.

I was 17 and I didn't realize that you had to be 21 to be in those clubs, because I'd already been working in the clubs [in Tulsa] for three years. I had to borrow IDs and union cards—the union had a deal that you couldn't work in the clubs unless you belonged to their local, and once you belonged to that local, you couldn't work for a year. So I had to borrow union cards and IDs, and I'd last until they got a new bouncer. I'd come to work, and he'd want to see my ID, and I'd already given it back to whomever I'd borrowed it from, so I'd lose that job. It was kind of rough.

Russell persevered, however, and the week he turned 21, "when I was legal to work in clubs," he got his first couple of studio sessions. "They just started doubling every week after that," he recalled, "and I quit playing in clubs."

Within a year, Russell was one of the top studio cats in L.A., a member of the first-call musicians who comprised the elite recording group known as the Wrecking Crew. He began to arrange as well. And he built a recording studio in his home, with both the house and its studio becoming a way station for Tulsa rockers—and the occasional non-Tulsan, like Arkansan Levon Helm, later a founding member of the Band, and the brilliant guitarist Jesse Ed Davis, a Norman native—eager to jump into the exploding West Coast music scene.

As the '60s rolled on, the baby boomers hit their teens. They had disposable incomes, and they wanted to spend at least part of that cash on their own kind of music, the music and musicians they were hearing on Top 40 radio and, by the mid-'60s, watching on TV shows like *Shindig*, *Hullabaloo*, and *Where the Action Is*. The recording industry was more than happy to feed the kids' insatiable entertainment appetites, and the Tulsa guys got in on the act, many of them thanks, in no small part, to Russell's increasing presence in the industry.

Many of the Tulsa musicians first contributed to the American rock-music scene by doing studio work—usually helped along by Russell—but they did other things as well. Jumpin' Jack Dunham signed with Imperial Records and cut several singles; Chuck Blackwell became the drummer for the Shindogs, the house band for the *Shindig* TV show; and several Tulsans became members of Gary Lewis and the Playboys. Others make up the band of major-label bluesman Taj Mahal, Jimmy Markham and fellow Tulsan Roger Tillison sang on a couple of major-label projects, and Markham recorded four sides for Capitol as the leader of Jimmy Markham and the Tulsa Rhythm Revue, which included Johnny Cale, Jesse Ed Davis, bassist Gary Gilmore and Jimmy Karstein. Russell himself became a studio kingpin, arranging, writing, and playing keyboards (and occasionally other instruments, including the bass on the Byrds' 1965 No. 1, "Mr. Tambourine Man") on tons of hit singles and albums. Gates also worked behind the scenes during the '60s in similar capacities, prior to forming the hit soft-rock group Bread in the late '60s, although his career path had already diverged from that of most of his fellow Tulsans, who were enjoying the rock 'n' roll lifestyle on the Coast. As his work as an early Tulsa rocker foreshadowed, Gates approached the business in a more reasoned, less hedonistic, way.

> "AS THE '60s ROLLED ON, THE BABY BOOMERS HIT THEIR TEENS. THEY HAD DISPOSABLE INCOMES, AND THEY WANTED TO SPEND AT LEAST PART OF THAT CASH ON THEIR OWN KIND OF MUSIC, THE MUSIC AND MUSICIANS THEY WERE HEARING ON TOP 40 RADIO AND, BY THE MID-'60s, WATCHING ON TV SHOWS LIKE SHINDIG, HULLABALOO, AND WHERE THE ACTION IS."

Once Johnny Cale rolled into town, he helped run Leon's home studio and worked at other studios, hustled club gigs, and took a couple of shots at recording a hit single himself. "In those days," he said with a laugh, "you could sell almost anything." While he didn't become a major recording presence until the early '70s, Cale recorded some intriguing material in the early '60s, including "Dick Tracy," a wacky ode to the comic-strip character created by fellow

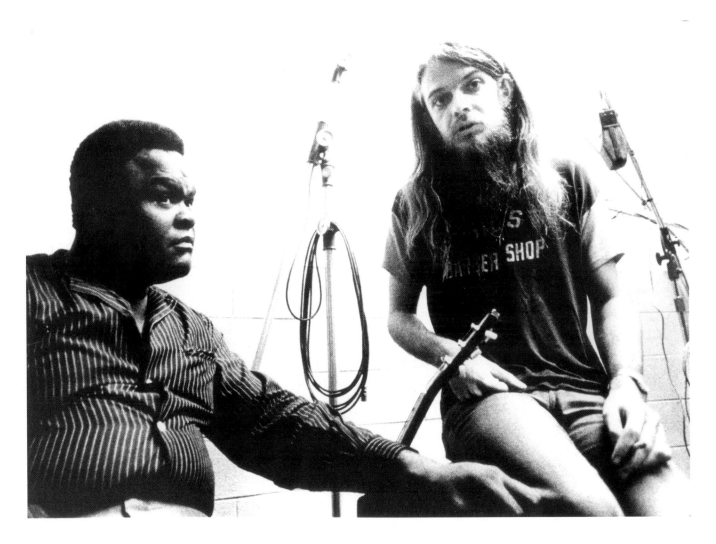

Freddie King and Leon Russell

Oklahoman Chester Gould.

Cale, of course, would see fame as J.J. Cale, not Johnny. It's been widely written that his name was Jean Jaques Cale, which makes some sense. But, according to Cale, that's based on an erroneous article penned by a foreign journalist many years ago. In fact, the name change had to do with another Johnny entirely. As Cale explained, it happened in the mid-'60s.

Me and Gary Sanders, who's passed away, and [bassist] Gary Gilmore were playing joints out in California, and we went out and auditioned for the Whisky A-Go-Go. It was the happenin' Hollywood place. Johnny Rivers had the gig there, and at the time he had a hit record out that he'd recorded down at that joint. So he was kind of big time and this joint was, to our viewpoint, Hollywood big time.

He [Rivers] was taking two nights off a week, and so the Joint's owner, Elmer Valentine, said, "We need somebody." So we went down there and auditioned. It was really a high-paying gig compared to all the other gigs in L.A. So the guy said, "Well, Johnny Cale's okay, but I'll give you the job if I can change your name to J.J."

I said, "Man, you give me a job, and you can call me anything you want to call me!" Because we were starving. I mean, we were eatin' popcorn and livin' funky.

So he said, "I'm going to change your name to J.J. and put it on the marquee on the two nights you're playing here." And I said, "Go right ahead, Jack."

That's what happened. My name's John W. Cale. But we just needed to work. I was looking for the money, because Hollywood's a rough deal.

Cale would continue to scuffle for a few more years, writing and performing songs in his uniquely laid-back style, before British rock star Eric Clapton discovered him and his songs, including the Cale-penned "After Midnight" and "Cocaine." Clapton's treatment of those numbers led to greater visibility for the somewhat reclusive Cale, who became a recording star in his own right and remains a major cult figure to this day.

His deep-groove, blues-based, deceptively simple-sounding music not only heavily influenced Clapton (and others), but became a major component of the classic Tulsa Sound as well.

Clapton was only one of the artists in the orbit of Leon Russell, whose career had escalated dramatically by the late 1960s. Poised on the brink of major stardom, he hit the tipping point as musical director of and performer on the Mad Dogs and Englishmen tour, a 43-piece rock-music revue designed to showcase raspy-voiced British vocalist Joe Cocker. The shows and subsequent records indeed did that for Cocker, but they also brought a lot of attention to Russell himself.

To understand the influence Russell—and, by extension, Tulsa—was having on the rock scene at the turn of the decade, all you have to do is take a look at the *Mad Dogs and Englishmen* documentary, which was reissued on DVD in 2006. There, you'll not only spot a lot of Tulsa musicians who were integral to the tour and its sound, but you'll also see an up-and-coming Russell, confident and in control, sure-handedly maneuvering Cocker and the rest of the players into a musical force different from anything heard before—unless, of course, you'd seen Russell and his cohorts jamming in Tulsa clubs or in his home studio on the West Coast. It was a sound that blended blues and rock 'n' roll and gospel, and even a little country music, all melding into something immediately recognizable but hard to categorize.

Although it's impossible to know exactly how much of an impact the Mad Dogs and Englishmen tour had on other rockers, and on the state of the music in general, it's safe to say that it opened a lot of ears. A Top 10 Cocker hit from 1970, reworking the old Top 40 Box Tops hit, "The Letter," was recorded live with Russell and a large backing group known as the Shelter People, giving a good idea of what Mad Dogs and Englishmen sounded like live.

Another 1970 radio hit, "God, Love And Rock & Roll," also captured that sound. That was only right, since the artists, Teegarden & Van Winkle, were drummer David Teegarden and keyboardist Skip "Van Winkle" Knape, a pair of Tulsans transplanted to Detroit. Well before that move, however, they'd been two of many Tulsans to accept Russell's hospitality on the West Coast. In a 1997 interview, Teegarden recalled those days.

We got together in L.A. and we were living at Leon's house and we didn't do much work, but that's when we kind of got into our recording career. Cale was running Leon's studio, in Leon's house. Cale came up every day and worked in the studio, and he got to recording us. We did a single as the Sunday Servants.

A cover of the 1955 R&B hit "Bo Diddley," the Sunday Servants' single didn't go anywhere. But several years later, "God, Love And Rock & Roll" made it to No. 22 on the Billboard magazine singles chart. Teegarden noted that it was heavily influenced by what Russell was doing with Mad Dogs and Englishmen.

Everybody we knew from Tulsa was on that gig, and Detroit was their first show. I remember that Leon and Denny Cordell had to rent an airplane to get the whole entourage from L.A. to Detroit and it cost 'em $20,000. They called us, said "c'm'on down," and it was like we were on the gig with 'em. We ended up on stage—I was playing tambourine—and we got real inspired because that band sounded so good. So we went home and started working on "God, Love And Rock & Roll."

In many ways, 1970 was the year of the Tulsa Sound, or at least Leon Russell's version of it. And not long after it grabbed the attention of listeners all over the world, he decided to bring it back home.

I moved back here [to Tulsa] and bought some property up on Grand Lake. That's where I was living at the time, and I think we just kind of opened an office here, because that's where I was. I'd been to California five or six times before that happened. I'd go out there and stay for six months or so and starve and get sick, and then I'd have to come back for a month or two to recuperate. So that Shelter thing—it seems to me it may have come along as

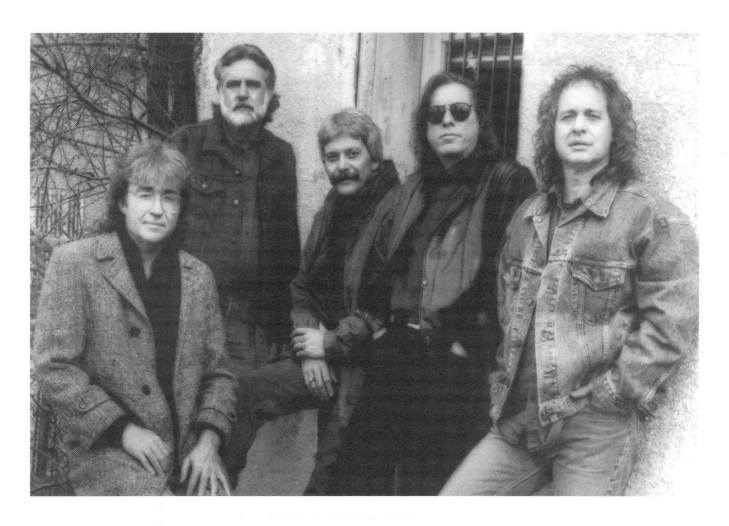

The Tractors, circa 1994: Walt Richmond, Casey Van Beek, Ron Getman, Jamie Oldaker, and Steve Ripley

long as 10 years after the first time I went out there. So I'd been out there a good little while when that happened.

—*Leon Russell*

During Leon Russell's '60s days as a major West Coast studio player, he'd hooked up with British producer Denny Cordell, which was how the whole Joe Cocker connection got started. Cocker had a hit with the Russell composition "Delta Lady," and then came the Mad Dogs and Englishmen tour and more Cocker hits.

The association with Cordell also brought a partnership. Together, they formed Shelter Records and took up residence in a stately old building near downtown Tulsa that had once housed the First Church of God. Converted into a recording studio, it became known, naturally enough, as the Church Studio.

Shelter Records signed a number of artists, including vocalist Phoebe Snow, rockers Tom Petty and the Heartbreakers (who did a significant amount of recording at Church Studio), and blues great Freddie King. Of course, Tulsans were well-represented on the roster as well. Cale signed with Shelter, as did younger guys Dwight Twilley and Phil Seymour (who cut the early version of Twilley's 1975 breakout hit "I'm on Fire" at the Church), and the R&B outfit the GAP Band, whose initials came from the north Tulsa streets Greenwood, Archer, and Pine.

Meanwhile, Russell had become a major star himself, hobnobbing with rock royalty like George Harrison and Bob Dylan. His move back to Tulsa catalyzed a heady period for the town's music scene—the clubs were full of backup singers, nationally known musicians, and members of British nobility, as well as the occasional superstar who'd blown into town to spend a few days hanging out with Russell and Cordell. Homegrown bands and vocalists popped up all over, with many of their members ultimately snagged by major touring acts. Eric Clapton was especially influenced by what he saw and heard from Tulsa, using bassist Carl Radle, drummer Jamie Oldaker and keyboardist Dick Sims in his band and recording J.J. Cale songs. Clapton's guitar style also changed following his exposure to the Tulsa Sound, becoming much more spare and laid-back. People credit that to Cale, which indeed may be true, but it's also true that at one point Clapton was listening a lot to Tulsa's Rockin' Jimmy Byfield and the Brothers of the Night, whose guitarist Steve Hickerson played in that manner as well. Clapton even recorded a Byfield tune, "Little Rachel."

When people think of the classic Tulsa Sound, then they think of that period in the early to mid-'70s, when Russell returned home and the city vibrated with music that sounded fresh and new and exciting. But as we've seen, the seed of that sound had been planted in the mid-1950s, by Russell and others. His return simply brought it up out of the Tulsa soil, where it flowered profusely for a few years, multiplying and trailing out well beyond the city limits of the town that gave it birth.

And now that we know when and how it happened, maybe it's time to take a look at what it is.

Well, I suppose there is [a Tulsa Sound], but you're talking to somebody that's in the middle of it. That's kind of like asking a fish about the properties of water. It's difficult to really know.
—*Leon Russell*

Every city of any size has its musicians who've

gone off and made something of themselves, whether as sidemen or stars, behind the scenes or in the spotlight. And at some point, anyone who chronicles a certain music scene has got to stand back, take a good hard look at things, and answer a difficult question: Is our scene *really* all that different, or did we just have a good bunch of people get out there and make some lasting noise in pop music?

The Tulsa Sound isn't as easy to pin down as western swing—which, after all, became its own musical genre. There are some who say there's no such thing as the Tulsa Sound. And there are others who say that the sound itself is more than one thing.

Bassist Gerald Goodwin, who played with just about all of the Tulsa Sound pioneers in the 1950s, including David Gates and the Accents, believes that the music is rooted in simplicity, a theory echoed by many of his contemporaries.

I think what they call the Tulsa Sound is more heavily based around the clubs—Johnny Cale, and Leon Russell, and Chuck Blackwell, and I'll brag a little and say myself. It was a hard-driving sound, a very clean crisp drum sound. All drummers wanted to be jazz drummers and play a lot of flourishes, but somehow, we just hit on the idea of keeping it simple. Somebody like Chuck would really drive a song, by just keeping it very simple on the ride cymbal and snare and bass, and the bass line to me was a little unique in that I felt like it should be pushed. It should stay on top of the beat. It gave a sort of tension to the music. It had a certain tightness to it.

Then, Leon sort of single-handedly put the keyboards into the picture. You could never hear the piano in any rock band. They didn't have amplification. But through his vision and his talent, he made that a big part of the sound, along with a good clean guitar by somebody like Cale. The Accents were more into socially acceptable music—music that was easy, danceable, and always meticulously played by David. There was the David crowd, and there was the Leon crowd. You see the music that David produced and performed [after Tulsa], and that came out of high school. You see the music Leon does, and that came out of the clubs. After they separated, they went very different ways, musically.

Emily Smith, a Russell friend and confidant for many years, has long maintained that the Tulsa Sound has to do with the space between notes, best exemplified by Cale and extending to trumpeter Chet Baker, who left his Oklahoma hometown of Yale for California in the '50s, becoming a leading light of the West Coast cool-jazz school. Perhaps unsurprisingly, he played several gigs in Tulsa with local musicians during the '70s.

Tulsa keyboardist and singer Larry Bell, who came along a little after the first wave of '50s

Tulsa rockers, echoed Smith's observations. "The main thing I learned from my elders," he said in a 2003 conversation, "is less is more. Period."

You don't sing everything. You don't play every note you know. You play from your heart, not from your fingers. You can play half a dozen notes at the right places, and not have to be Segovia, and really knock some people flat. That's one trick that you learned—play the right note at the right time, and know when not *to play. That's the key.*

Veteran keyboardist Rocky Frisco, who was known as Rocky Curtiss when he played during the first wave of the Tulsa Sound—and who still tours with J.J. Cale—added these comments in a 2003 interview.

Cale said it better than anybody. He said he really wanted to be able to play the blues, and wanted to be able to play the new rock 'n' roll, and he was trying to play like Chuck Berry and all these people. But he said he couldn't quite do it, so he made up something on his own. So, basically, the Tulsa Sound is a bunch of people who couldn't play the blues trying to play the blues. We all loved the blues, but we couldn't play it. We all pretended *we could.*

In addition to that laid-back blues-based approach, however, there's a kind of shuffle beat that's also associated with the Tulsa Sound. Second-generation Tulsa Sound figure Don White put it this way in his "Tulsa Shuffle No. 1":

They like the blues up in Chicago
Country in Tennessee
The honky-tonks in Texas
That's good enough for me
They like it hard and loud in Detroit
California's got a brand-new sound
But when you're back in Tulsa
You gotta lay that shuffle down
(Darn Write Music, BMI)

The multi-platinum-selling 1994 debut album by the Tractors, a Tulsa-based outfit full of first-tier T-town musicians and headed by singer-songwriter-guitarist Steve Ripley—a bridge, as we'll see later, between the Tulsa Sound and the Red Dirt movement of the '90s—contains its own "Tulsa Shuffle," a song different from White's that nonetheless celebrates the same kind of music. (And there's a third "Tulsa Shuffle" out there as well, written and recorded in 1969 by former T-towner Elvin Bishop, a noted bluesman who didn't actually begin his music career until after he left Tulsa for Chicago in 1959.)

Interestingly enough, it's the most famous song from that first Tractors album, an upbeat tune called "Baby Likes to Rock It," (which was a hit on the national country charts), that David Gates believes best exemplifies a major part of Tulsa's classic Sound.

If you examine the rhythm of that record, it's what

we were doing in Tulsa clubs. Even today, when I get around California musicians and East Coast musicians, it's hard for them to grasp this tight shuffle. That became the foundation of the Tulsa Sound. When we played shuffles, we would imitate certain shuffles and certain straight-eighth things, but we had this little groove of our own.

The straight-eight beat, he added, is all eighth notes, as in Chuck Berry's classic "Johnny B. Goode," while a shuffle beat is a dotted eighth and a sixteenth note, as in Berry's "Sweet Little Sixteen."

The way the Tulsa guys shuffled is that we tightened it up and interpreted it slightly different. "Baby Likes to Rock It" is a tighter groove. It's between the straight-eighths and the shuffle, and it's the one people [outside of Tulsa] have a hard time with. But if you listen to that record and then put on "Sweet Little Sixteen," you'll hear the difference.

In a recent article for the online publication *Tulsa Today*, writer-musician Jim Downing (aka James McMaster Downing) explored several theories about what makes the Tulsa Sound unique, concluding that part of it "probably has to do with the size of Tulsa."

This is not a big city, and it's easier for musicians to get together. High school rivalries and race mean nothing to musicians. In a bigger city, it may be harder to connect with like-minded individuals and find a place to practice. I attended an all-day benefit in Chicago a few years ago with 23 of that city's working bands. These were not amateurs; I saw most of them listed in the paper, playing at popular clubs. To my utter shock, of the 23, I heard only one band that could get a job in Tulsa.

That's a valid observation, and it's just as valid when applied to the pioneers of the Tulsa Sound. If Russell and Gates and Jack Dunham hadn't known the musicians from Tulsa who began streaming to the West Coast in the '60s, it's unlikely they would've offered shelter and encouragement—or at least as much of it as they did. In part because of the manageable size of the rock 'n' roll scene in Tulsa then, all of these singers and instrumentalists knew one another. Most of them had even played on stage in bands together. Dunham believes that the familiarity the players had with each other is directly responsible for the Tulsa Sound.

I think it all originated back in the time we were playing, and we interchanged musicians so much. Like [bassist Ralph] Brummett would bring his riffs to the stage, and Chuck Blackwell would bring his drum parts; Doug Cunningham would play piano, and he'd be different from Rocky Curtiss, who was different from Leon. So everybody brought their own takes on how they would play a song.

Of course, it didn't hurt that Gates, Russell, and Cale came out of that group, all becoming music stars and influential artists as well, while many of their Tulsa rock 'n' roll contemporaries also had their impact on the national scene, either from their session work or as members of major-label recording acts. Tulsa players became, for instance, integral parts of the bands of Bob Seger, Eric Clapton, Bonnie Raitt, Gary Lewis, Taj Mahal and Delaney & Bonnie, to name a few.

So, certainly, the relatively small size of the hometown music scene in the '50s, '60s and '70s had a lot to do with the Tulsa Sound, but that scene was also big enough to be fractured by runaway egos, differences of musical opinion, and the psychic fallout from real or imagined slights and injuries. Musicians, after all, are among the most thin-skinned of all artists, and it doesn't take much of a conflict to cause a band to crumble and float away like ashes in a prairie fire. Certainly, there were grudges nursed and enemies made during the pioneering days of the Tulsa Sound, but there was also a camaraderie and sense of brotherhood that held them together, just as those qualities had carried the Oklahoma City Blue Devils and the Bob and Johnnie Lee Wills groups through some challenging times over plenty of rough patches.

All musicians from a certain time and place have shared experiences and acquaintances, but the Tulsa Sound folks—in the true spirit of Oklahoma—seem to have taken that to another level. More than a half-century after the first wave of Tulsa musicians began interacting with one another on local stages, there's still that feeling of extended family among them, that Depression-era idea of the importance, and responsibility, each person had for taking care of others, and the notion that no matter your circumstances, you weren't any better than your neighbor. J.J. Cale saw this manifested in the way the Tulsa bands worked when one of the musicians had to bow out of a job.

With the Tulsa guys, it was funny. The bandleader would choose who was going to play, but if the drummer couldn't make it, if he had a better-paying gig on the same night, the bandleader wouldn't hire somebody else. The drummer would get somebody. If you had to bow out of a gig, it was an unspoken responsibility that you got somebody to cut the gig, so you wouldn't let the bandleader down. It seems like there was more of that [in Tulsa] than I've ever seen anywhere else. That was the Tulsa deal. Everybody was interchangeable.

Occasionally, that responsibility didn't just have to do with playing. It had to do with stepping aside and giving the job to someone better suited for it. Apparently, Leon Russell took that attitude with him to L.A., where, in 1963, he found himself working on a session for another Tulsan, western-swing great Leon McAuliffe. The steel-guitarist and bandleader was at Capitol Records, recording an album of pop standards that would be released by the label later that year as *The Dancin'est Band Around.*

In 1989, Russell friend, discographer and occasional concert promoter, Steve Todoroff interviewed McAuliffe about that record. "I thought it odd," Todoroff wrote in recent correspondence, "that Russell only had one song listed for that session, so I contacted Leon McAuliffe in March, 1989 at the college where he was teaching [Rogers State in Claremore, OK], and he told me the following:

Leon Russell did play on one of my sessions, a song called "I Fall to Pieces" on the Capitol Records instrumental album I produced. He came up to me after one song and said, "I'm not playing the style of piano that you need for this record. I've heard some of your piano players and I can't play like that." We got Billy Livert from Nashville to play on the rest of the sessions, but I always admired Leon for what he did that day.

That seems like a good place to end this chapter on the Tulsa Sound, with a revealing interchange between two of the most important figures in Oklahoma's music. They came from two different eras, and helped create and popularize two different musical styles, but a pro like Russell could easily have played his way through the album, taken the paycheck, and gone on to the next gig, with no one any wiser.

Was Russell motivated to do what he did in any way because McAuliffe was another Okie—and, indeed, a Tulsa music figure whose Cimarron Ballroom had been a part of Tulsa's early rock 'n' roll scene? Maybe so. But whatever his reasons, Russell's honest admission of his unsuitability for the job, and his stepping aside to let someone better for McAuliffe's sound take over, reinforces Cale's observation about individual band member's' responsibilities to the rest of the group.

So, whether the Tulsa Sound is best identified by Cale's deep groove, Russell's big gospel and R&B sound, or the tight shuffle Gates cited—or all three—its origins were rooted as much in the musicians' character, camaraderie and care for one another as it was in what they were playing. For that reason, as much as any other, you could shoot an arrow through the Oklahoma City Blue Devils, through Bob and Johnnie Lee Wills and the rest of Oklahoma's western swingers, through Woody Guthrie—and hit a bull's-eye right in the heart of the Tulsa Sound.

5

CHAPTER FIVE

THE BIGGEST COUNTRY MUSIC AGENCY IN THE WORLD

FROM about '75 to '82, when we had all the big stars, we did more business than all the booking agencies in Nashville combined. At one time, we did more than 400 fair dates in a year.
—Jim Halsey

In a music career that spans parts of seven decades, Jim Halsey's been a booking agent, manager, producer, promoter, and record-label executive, among other things. So instead of stacking all those nouns in front of his name, it's probably best to simply tag him with the label he prefers: "impresario."

Halsey was a high school student in Independence, Kansas, when he first became familiar with that term. It was the main title of a book he picked to read and report on for a class assignment, and as he related in a book he co-wrote with this author, *How to Make It in the Music Business* (HAWK Publishing/Halsey Books, 2000), running onto the story of a famed internationally known promoter and producer changed his life forever.

The book I chose was a biography called Impresario: A Memoir of Sol Hurok *(Random House, 1946).* Once I began reading it, I couldn't put it down. During his many years in show business, Sol Hurok presented nearly every type of stage attraction, specializing in bringing talent from the Soviet Union and other parts of Eastern Europe to the United States. His life had been full of glamour, talented artists, events that required creative sales and marketing, and even a certain amount of risk. What could be better for me? All through school I had been selling something. So why not sell music and entertainment?

Determined to become, as he put it in his book, "the impresario of southeastern Kansas," Halsey began by booking Tulsa-based western-swing figure Leon McAuliffe and his band into an auditorium in downtown Independence. Wandering around the streets of his hometown the night of the show, Halsey saw a line forming at the box office an hour before the band was to perform. That line presaged a full house, as well as the beginning of a long, full career for its fledgling promoter.

"That was my entry into show business," Halsey wrote. "I loved the music. I loved the excitement of seeing a promotion work. I loved the happiness on people's faces when they left, saying, 'Good dance, Jim,' or 'Good music, Jim,' or 'What a good time, Jim.' That night, I knew I was in show business to stay."

The year was 1949. Halsey had just turned 19. And a few years later, he'd be McAuliffe's booking agent, expanding the bandleader's territory beyond the Southwest and Midwest, where he was already well-established.

(Perhaps this is a good place to explain the difference between a booking agent, also known as simply an agent; a manager; and a promoter or producer. It's the agent's job to sell talent, to book an act with a promoter or producer—two terms that are pretty much interchangeable. The agent sells the act to the promoter, and the promoter then arranges for and promotes the show, hoping to make a profit. The manager takes care of an act's business, which may include record deals, corporate sponsorships, day-to-day expenses, and career planning, among other things. Sometimes, a person can be both agent and promoter, as Halsey was with western-swing star Hank Thompson for several years, or manager and agent. The point here is that the three jobs—agent, manager, and promoter—are all distinct and separate, even though you can sometimes find people who do all of them under the same roof, as was the case with the Jim Halsey Company during its years in Oklahoma.)

In addition to booking McAuliffe, Halsey soon began working with another western-swing star, Hank Thompson—a Texan who, you'll remember from an earlier chapter, had relocated to Oklahoma City. It could be seen as a swap of western-swing stars between not just the two states, but two cities as well. Thompson, originally from Waco, had been based in Dallas with his band, the Brazos Valley Boys, just before moving to OKC and getting established in the Trianon Ballroom. That's the same place Bob Wills and his Texas Playboys had called home before heading south to Dallas and a fabulous new hall Wills had built called the Bob Wills Ranch House.

Thompson moved to Oklahoma in 1950. Not coincidentally, that's the same year he met Jim Halsey. "In May 1950, Hank met a second crucial player in his blossoming organization," wrote Rich Kienzle in *Southwest Shuffle*. "Twenty-year-old Jim Halsey of Independence, Kansas, was still attending Independence Junior College when he started booking shows at the local Memorial Hall. The kid's able handling of Hank's Kansas and Oklahoma tours impressed both Hank and [Brazos Valley Boys bandleader Billy] Gray."

"I told Hank that Bob was moving out of the Trianon, and I thought we could get in there and get a radio show, maybe even a television show," said Halsey in a recent conversation.

His responsibilities with Thompson increasing, Halsey moved to Oklahoma City, setting up his office there on the first day of 1952. That's when he officially became Thompson's manager and agent. A few months later, Capitol Records

> **"THE POINT HERE IS THAT THE THREE JOBS—AGENT, MANAGER, AND PROMOTER—ARE ALL DISTINCT AND SEPARATE, EVEN THOUGH YOU CAN SOMETIMES FIND PEOPLE WHO DO ALL OF THEM UNDER THE SAME ROOF, AS WAS THE CASE WITH THE JIM HALSEY COMPANY DURING ITS YEARS IN OKLAHOMA."**

released Thompson's "Wild Side of Life," which became a giant hit for the Texas transplant and his band. The television show came along, too, that same eventful year. Called *The Big Red Shindig*, it aired every Saturday afternoon over Oklahoma City's WKY-TV, sponsored by a local furniture outlet called the Big Red Warehouse.

A year or so later, a teenager from Maude, who was living in the city with her family and attending Capitol Hill High School, snagged her own show on radio station KLPR. Wanda Jackson sang unadorned country music in her 15-minute program, and pretty soon she'd attracted Thompson's attention. Jackson acknowledged his influence on her and her career in a 1985 interview.

I'm his protégé. We were both living in Oklahoma City at the time, and I was singing on a local station, doing a radio show every day with just me and my guitar. One day, he heard me and invited me down to sing with his band, which was the biggest thrill of my life because he was my idol. Later, when I began to record, I recorded a lot of stuff at his house. He had a studio built in at the time. I'm sure he was also instrumental in getting me my contract with Capitol Records.

Before Capitol, however, Thompson helped the youngster get on the Decca label, where she recorded a duet with his bandleader, Billy Gray, called "You Can't Have My Love." It became a Top 10 hit on the national hillbilly-music charts, as they were known then, at just about the same time Jackson graduated from high school.

In 1955, the year Jackson got her diploma, Halsey was finishing a two-year stint as an Army draftee. Somehow, even while serving his country, he'd managed to hold onto his management and booking gigs with Thompson. Once discharged, he returned to Oklahoma City and was soon working with Jackson as well. They signed a deal that gave Halsey her exclusive representation, the same sort of deal he had with Thompson. Her subsequent signing with Capitol Records, on the strength of the sides she'd cut for Decca, put both of Halsey's artists on the same record label. Thompson had been with Capitol since 1948—he'd be a member of Capitol's recording-talent roster for nearly two decades.

Jackson, meanwhile, found herself on tour in a package show that included Elvis Presley, whose ascent to superstardom had already begun. They had a sweet romance—which she beguilingly described in a spoken-word track on her 2006 tribute disc, "I Remember Elvis"—and Presley convinced her to try her hand at the new kind of music that was making him more famous by the day. Her father and road manager, Tom Jackson, agreed with Presley, as Jackson recalled in a recent conversation.

Elvis and my daddy wore me down. My daddy

told me that the young people were starting to buy records. Before that, you know, adults bought the records, and that's why we all stayed in country music, because that's what the adults were buying.

Then, Elvis came along and turned everything upside down. None of us knew what was going on. We were just trying to hold on for dear life. And Elvis said, "If you get into this rockabilly, this rock 'n' roll, you'll sell a lot more records."

So, she started recording—and sometimes writing—scorching rockabilly numbers like "Mean, Mean Man," "Fujiyama Mama" and "Hot Dog! That Made Him Mad," records that still pack a considerable wallop a half-century later. It's that late-'50s work that have earned her the title of the First Lady of Rockabilly and attracted the attention of such musical heavyweights as Elvis Costello, who's one of many campaigning for her induction into the Rock and Roll Hall of Fame.

The fact is, however, that at the time those songs were a tough sell. As she remembered in a 2004 interview, "I had a hard time getting accepted by the people buying records. They had barely accepted Elvis and Jerry Lee Lewis, and when I came out shouting and swinging like those guys, they said, 'Whoa. Let's put *her* over in the corner for a while.'"

There were exceptions. As Carney and Foley note in their *Oklahoma Music Guide*, "Fujiyama Mama" became a huge hit in—perhaps not surprisingly—the country whose highest mountain gave the song its name, leading to "a sensational tour of Japan in 1959 with thousands of fans greeting her at every stop in the two-month tour." Her band for the trip came from Oklahoma as well. An integrated band, it included white vocalist and bandleader

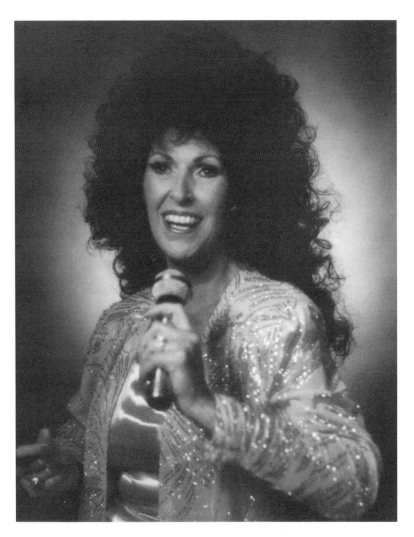

Wanda Jackson

Roy Clark

Bobby Poe, a Vinita native who'd later become a successful country-music promoter, and black piano player Al Downing of Lenapah. As Big Al Downing, he'd later see some success as an R&B artist in the '60s and early '70s before changing to country music and charting such hits as "Mr. Jones" and "Touch Me (Then I'll Be Your Fool Once More)." Downing's piano is also heard on "Let's Have a Party," the only one of Jackson's rockabilly rave-ups to make the national Top 40.

By the time "Let's Have a Party" peaked on the charts in August 1960, Jackson was in the middle of a year-long engagement at the Golden Nugget in Las Vegas, a booking negotiated by Halsey. Before that gig had even begun, however, Jackson had taken on a new band and hired a new front man who would later become the flagship artist of the Jim Halsey Company, and a major international star who still shines today.

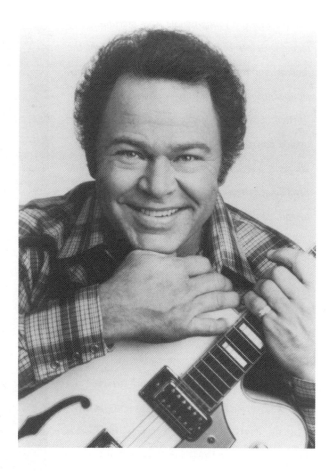

Hank Thompson introduced Wanda to the world, and after Wanda made it, she helped usher in another new star, one who would become one of my biggest stars and dearest friends...

Wanda described him as a multi-talented musician, singer, and showman. When I saw him play his first concert with her, I saw that she'd been conservative in her description. He turned out to be all she'd said he was—and a whole lot more. To this day, I have not seen a greater talent.

His name? Roy Clark.

—*Jim Halsey,*
FROM HOW TO MAKE IT IN THE MUSIC BUSINESS

A Virginia native raised in the Washington,

D.C. area, Roy Linwood Clark grew up playing guitar, banjo and mandolin, and was accomplished enough as a musician to begin earning money as a teenager. His first paying job was with his dad's square-dance band, where he received two dollars for a night's work. Preferring music to school, he dropped out before getting his diploma and began playing the clubs around the D.C. area. That led to tours with country-music package shows, one of them headed by Hank Williams. By 1959, when Wanda Jackson first encountered him in a Washington club, Clark had won a national banjo competition; performed at the Grand Ole Opry; played with stars like Jimmy Dean, Red Foley, Grandpa Jones and Ernest Tubb; and honed his entertainment chops playing a variety of musical styles in various D.C. nightspots.

Like Jackson, Halsey was knocked out the first time he saw Clark on stage.

"Even in 1959," Halsey wrote, "fronting someone else's band, Roy had 'superstardom' written all over his performance. He connected with his audience like nobody I had ever seen."

Clark and Halsey connected as well. Going out on his own after the Vegas engagement, with Halsey as his manager and agent, Clark quickly became a touring star and recording artist. Just as Thompson had helped Jackson get on Capitol Records, Jackson recommended Clark to the same label. By 1963, he had his first Top 10 country hit, "The Tips of My Fingers," which made some noise on the pop charts as well. It was that appeal to audiences both within and beyond the country-music mainstream that fueled Roy Clark's major stardom—he was a country act that people who didn't know anything about country music could enjoy, an affable entertainer whose down-home comedic persona complemented his lightning fingers and soulful singing voice.

The same year "Tips of My Fingers" hit, Clark made his first appearance on *The Tonight Show with Johnny Carson*, where he would return for years as one of Carson's favorite guests and fill-in hosts. He'd do many other television shows as well, but his major and most lasting impression in the medium came with his decades-spanning

> **"HE WAS A COUNTRY ACT THAT PEOPLE WHO DIDN'T KNOW ANYTHING ABOUT COUNTRY MUSIC COULD ENJOY, AN AFFABLE ENTERTAINER WHOSE DOWN-HOME COMEDIC PERSONA COMPLEMENTED HIS LIGHTNING FINGERS AND SOULFUL SINGING VOICE."**

stint as co-host (with Buck Owens) of *Hee Haw*. A combination of music and comedy sketches, *Hee Haw* began life in 1969 as a hillbilly version of the then-hugely popular comedy series *Rowan & Martin's Laugh-In*. Going into syndication after a couple of years as a network offering, it outlasted the show that inspired it by almost two decades, finally expiring in 1992. Clark stayed with it all the way. (Another Oklahoman, Tulsa-based character actor and comedian Gailard Sartain, was also a longtime member of the *Hee Haw* cast.)

When Jim Halsey moved his base of operations to Tulsa in 1971, Thompson had already relocated to nearby Sand Springs. It took Clark a couple more years to become an Oklahoman, although, as he recalled in a 1988 interview, he'd been thinking about it for a while.

Jim Halsey...was really knocked out with the city [of Tulsa]. I lived back in Maryland at the time, and he told me if I lived in Tulsa I could have an additional 20 days at home with the same schedule. Because then, I was looking at starting a tour by going from Maryland to California, so I'd lose a day there, and then the tour would end in California, and I'd lose a day coming home.

Roy and his wife, Barbara, found a house in Tulsa a year or two after Halsey established his company there, but they didn't actually relocate until 1976. Or, rather, Barbara and their furniture relocated, since Clark was across the world in the midst of a tour of the Soviet Union, which still stands as one of his and Halsey's most spectacular accomplishments. Accompanied by the Oak Ridge Boys, another of Halsey's clients, Clark and his band, Rodney Lay and the Wild West, did eighteen sold-out shows in the USSR—which, at the time, reigned as America's nemesis in the Cold War.

Halsey described the genesis of that tour in his book:

In May 1974, an event took shape that would change my life.

Roy Clark was headlining in Las Vegas, doing one of his two-week engagements at the Frontier Hotel. Late one afternoon, he and I were sitting around in his hotel suite, watching the evening news, when a segment appeared about a group of Soviet dignitaries at the Seattle World's Fair. They were on an official visit to America, and the TV interviewer asked them if there was any place in the U. S. not on their official itinerary that they'd really like to see.

"Yes," immediately answered Alexi Stepunin, the delegates' leader. "We had hoped to visit Las Vegas, but it was not included in our trip."

I think Roy and I both got the idea simultaneously.

"Roy," I said, "let's invite them to see your show, as your guests."

The delegation quickly got that invitation, the State Department approved, and that was the beginning of the process that led Clark, the Oak Ridge Boys and Halsey to the Soviet Union. Although that trip would be a great success, Halsey wrote that he wasn't sure how it was going to turn out when he looked at the audience assembled in a hall in Riga, Latvia, for the first Soviet show.

The concert began with a cold audience, and the well-below-zero temperature outside had little to do with it. You could feel the attitude rising off the entire opening-night crowd. Okay, Americans, they seemed to be saying, **prove to us how good you are. Make us enjoy it…**

What happened next is impossible to describe adequately. As I stood backstage watching, Roy came out and began the show. Within 30 seconds, he'd changed the entire audience's mood from cold, impassive hostility to warm, loving friendship. A few more minutes into the show, and he was getting the kind of reception and acceptance these Soviet citizens would've given their country's biggest hero. He was not only entertaining them; he had won them over!

Clark returned for a 12-concert tour of Leningrad and Moscow in 1988. By that time, the country was much different, thanks to the policy of *glasnost*, or openness, instituted by Soviet leader Mikhail Gorbachev in the mid-'80s. Gorbachev, in fact, had mentioned Clark as one of the entertainers he'd like to see in his country.

"What really started this trip was when Mr. Gorbachev, at the first of the year, said he wanted to increase the exchange of American artists," said Clark a couple of months before the tour began. "And he personally invited Roy Clark, Billy Joel, and Stevie Wonder.

"This article was carried by UPI or the AP, one of 'em, and you see these things every now and

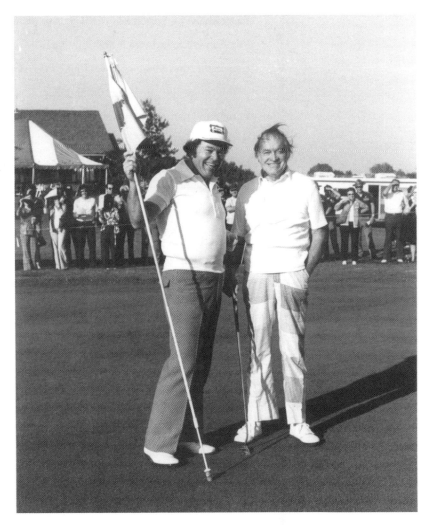

Roy Clark & Bob Hope

then, when some overzealous PR person plants 'em. So we checked into it and found out it had come right from Moscow. It was legit."

This time, the trip—dubbed the Roy Clark Friendship Tour—was sponsored in great part by private donations. The fundraising kicked off at a $100-a-plate dinner in Nashville, where Halsey Company clients mingled with special guest Bob Hope and other dignitaries, including then-Tennessee Senator Al Gore, who made this comment from the dais: "If every member of the [Soviet] Politboro would've grown up watching *Hee Haw*, the world would be a safer and saner place."

Clark and Halsey collaborated on a number of other notable projects, many of them back in their adopted hometown of Tulsa. That's where the Roy Clark Star Nights and Roy Clark Celebrity Golf Tournaments ran in the '70s and '80s, events chock-full of big name acts that cumulatively raised well over a million dollars for Tulsa's Children's Medical Center. Those were the golden days of the Jim Halsey Company in Oklahoma, when the client list included, in addition to Clark and Hank Thompson—who were also Halsey business partners—such famous artists as Waylon Jennings, Merle Haggard, the Oak Ridge Boys, Tammy Wynette, Clint Black, Conway Twitty, the Judds, Ronnie Milsap, Mel and Pam Tillis, Roy Orbison, and Dwight Yoakam, plus many others. Oklahoma's Reba McEntire was also represented by the agency, as were non-country acts like big-band legend Woody Herman, soul-music godfather James Brown, and Tulsa Sound pioneer and rock superstar Leon Russell.

In the late '70s, Halsey was the executive producer of a couple of well-received albums: *Reunion*, a disc that reunited western-swing great Johnnie Lee Wills with his favorite sidemen, and *Makin' Music*, a spirited teaming of Roy Clark and the unclassifiable guitarist and vocalist Clarence "Gatemouth" Brown. The former was released on Flying Fish Records, the latter on MCA, although both were produced by Steve Ripley, who would eventually find multi-platinum success with his own band, the Tractors.

A few years later, Halsey's impulse to make albums led to Churchill Records, a Tulsa-based company helmed by Halsey's son Sherman, who is now a noted director of videos and television shows, including a couple of Tim McGraw network specials. In its relatively short life, Churchill released discs by Hank Thompson and Roy Clark, as well as one from well-known Tulsa vocalist Debbie Campbell and a couple of singles by a Tulsa-based country singer named Ronnie Dunn—who, after joining Louisiana's Kix Brooks, would become a part of the most successful duo in country music history, Brooks & Dunn.

Although Churchill landed a distribution deal with the giant MCA Records, the Tulsa outfit had to deal with the usual problems small labels have in making the national country-music charts. The most successful Churchill artist when it came to airplay was a young lady named Cindy Hurt, whose singles "Don't Come Knockin'" and "Talk to Me Loneliness" both hit the Top 30, a ranking good enough to get her named *Billboard* magazine's Number One New Female Country Singles Artist for 1982.

For several years, the Halsey Company billed itself as the biggest country music agency in the world, a label that remains undisputed. Under the company's umbrella, scores of people worked in booking, production, recording, and personal management with acts that ranged from huge to virtually unknown. The influence of the massive outfit on the country-music scene during those years, and beyond, extended not only across America but across the planet. Halsey firmly believed, and still believes, that music is a powerful force for changing the world. Many of his projects during this time—including the Roy Clark USSR trips, the Oak Ridge Boys' involvement with financing the drilling of water wells in a drought-stricken portion of Africa, his support of international music festivals, and even the benefit component of the annual Roy Clark events—put that belief into action.

As the old axiom tells us, nothing lasts forever, and in 1987 Halsey moved the bulk of his agency to Nashville, where it merged, three years later, with the William Morris Agency. He maintained an office in the Tulsa area, however, and—like Clark—continues to make his home there. While Halsey concentrates more on consulting and teaching these days, he still manages the Oak Ridge Boys, a relationship that's lasted almost three decades. And he maintains his sharp eye for new talent. He was, for instance, one of the first music-industry figures to see the potential of Hanson, the Tulsa pop-rock group that had such a huge run in the late '90s. Halsey predicted stardom for them when they were still the Hansons, playing local gigs like Tulsa's Mayfest.

Recently, Halsey noted that while Independence, Kansas is his hometown, "I've always called Tulsa my spiritual home." His comments show, once again, the unmistakable connection of Oklahoma's music scenes, and how one generation's music leads into another.

I was born and raised in Independence, which is only 85 miles north of Tulsa, and I'd come down here and see [evangelist] Oral Roberts, and wrestling matches, and Bob Wills. It must've been 1939 or '40 when I first went to see Bob Wills.

He was at the old Philtower Building then, and my uncle brought me down. He and [KVOO owner and oilman] W.G. Skelly had some joint business ventures, and I remember going in to see Bob Wills with my uncle holding one of my hands and W.G. Skelly holding the other. That was such an impressionable time for me.

Unlike most of the other figures in this book, Halsey came to the music business not as a performer, but as a businessman. Perhaps that's the reason why he has a different take on how Oklahoma—and, specifically, Tulsa—influenced him and his work.

The reason I've always felt akin to Tulsa was the entrepreneurial spirit. It's there because of the oil business. The town's imbued with it—those guys making deals in the lobby of the Mayo Hotel, or the Tulsa Hotel, carrying their leases around in their hip pockets. I felt a kinship with that energy, that entrepreneurial, promoter-type spirit those guys had. It's out there, that excitement.

On the other hand, the artist most identified with Halsey during those heady years—a performer who's made such an impact on popular culture that a Tulsa elementary school was named after him in 1977—echoed what so many other Oklahoma musicians have noted about the brotherhood and sense of community in the state. Although no longer represented by Halsey, Roy Clark's home and office—and heart—remain in Tulsa.

"I like Tulsa because I didn't have to change anything when I moved here," he said in a 1988 conversation. "See, I was born down in the southwestern part of Virginia, a very rural area, where people know people and you depend on people. I found that same thing here in Oklahoma.

"So I don't have to change my thinking," he concluded. "As far as people knowing people and doing for each other, that's all right here in Tulsa."

JOHN WOOLEY

6
CHAPTER SIX
OKLAHOMA TAKES NASHVILLE

THESE days, if you're in Nashville and you say that you're from Oklahoma, it helps. People take notice, that's for sure.
— country star Joe Diffie, 1991

Even back when most of the country called it by names like "hillbilly" and "cowboy," Oklahomans were involved in country music in major ways. Although his work owed as much to Dixieland jazz and pop as it did to anything else, Bob Wills wore that hillbilly tag throughout much of his career, as did his fellow western swingers. On the cowboy side of things, exemplified by the singing heroes of the musical B-westerns, the state contributed a couple of guys who hit the very top: western-movie superstar Gene Autry, a Texas native who grew up in Oklahoma and got his first big break on Tulsa's KVOO (later, of course, the home of Bob Wills), where he was billed as "Oklahoma's Yodeling Cowboy"; and Tim Spencer, born in Missouri but raised in Picher, who was a founding member of and major songwriter for the Sons of the Pioneers, who first achieved prominence in the 1930s and are still the yardstick by which any cowboy-music group is measured. A third B-western star and recording artist, Jimmy Wakely, was an Arkansas native who grew up in various Oklahoma towns. Wakely played regular radio jobs on both Oklahoma City's WKY and Tulsa's KVOO before heading for California and hitting it big–with the help of Autry, who gave him his first national break by putting Wakely's trio on his network radio show, *Melody Ranch*.

In the 1950s, as the genre began shedding its "hillbilly" tag for an image that was a bit more cosmopolitan, and Nashville began its ascendancy as the country music capital of the world, a steady stream of Okies continued to find employment as singers and songwriters, with some becoming significant stars. Oklahoma City native Molly Bee, for instance, was a big draw in the '50s and early '60s, thanks in great part to her TV and movie exposure. The irrepressible singer-songwriter Roger Miller, a Texas native who grew up in Erick, poured his off-trail sense of humor and manic personality into crossover-hit records like "Dang Me" and "King of the Road," becoming a big-name performer in the bargain. Pauls Valley native Jean Shepherd maintained a country chart presence from the '50s well into the '70s, and Oklahoma-linked acts like Cal Smith, Henson Cargill, Bonnie Owens, Carl Belew, Billy Parker, Jody Miller, Tommy Overstreet and Norma Jean also made their own marks with country-radio listeners within that time.

Some Oklahoma recording artists soared all the way to the top spot, including Gans native Smith—with his wonderfully self-righteous "The Lord Knows I'm Drinkin'" (1973) as well as the tough tear-jerker "Country Bumpkin" (1974)—and Oklahoma City's Cargill, whose 1967 hard-bitten social-commentary single "Skip A Rope" found an audience not only on country radio but at pop outlets as well. It should also be noted that two huge figures in '50s pop music, Claremore's Patti Page and Dougherty's Kay Starr, often recorded country songs and had plenty of success with country audiences. Page's "Tennessee Waltz," released in 1950, hit the top spot on both the pop and hillbilly charts, on its way to becoming one of the bestselling singles of all time, while Starr's 1950 version of Pee Wee King's country hit "Bonaparte's Retreat" became one of the biggest records of her long career.

But all of that, impressive though it may be, could hardly prepare an observer for what happened in the early '90s, when Oklahoma acts took over Nashville.

That may sound like hyperbole. It's not.

Consider this: In 1991, when the Nashville-based Country Music Association celebrated its 25th year of giving awards to the top names in the industry, the list of potential winners was dominated by Norman's Vince Gill, with six nominations, and Tulsa native Garth Brooks, with five. The contenders for the top award of the night, Entertainer of the Year, included Brooks, Gill, and Chockie's Reba McEntire–who also hosted the show. When the dust cleared, Brooks had won the big one, along with taking Album of the Year (*No Fences*), Single of the Year ("Friends in Low Places") and Music Video of the Year ("The Thunder Rolls," a controversial video that depicted domestic abuse). Gill had snagged Male Vocalist of the Year, and, with Grove songwriter turned record-company executive Tim DuBois, Song of the Year ("When I Call Your Name"), the CMA's top songwriting award. Gill had also picked up a third trophy for Vocal Event of the Year, acknowledging his work on the single "Restless" as a member of the one-off group Mark O'Conner and the Nashville Cats.

The next year, the same three acts were up for CMA's Entertainer of the Year again, along with non-Okies Alan Jackson and Travis Tritt. (Each category had five finalists.) And once again, Brooks won it. Gill also repeated as Male Vocalist of the Year–besting two Tulsa natives, Brooks and Joe Diffie, as well as Jackson and Tritt.

Nineteen-ninety-two was also the year that a duo put together by Grove's DuBois (then the vice president and general manager of Arista Nashville) first hit the short list of CMA nominees. Brooks & Dunn were Kix Brooks, a singer-songwriter from Louisiana, and Ronnie Dunn, a seasoned club performer from Texas who'd been honing his chops in Tulsa-area clubs and honky-tonks since the early '70s. After being paired by DuBois as a songwriting and then a recording team, the two lost the 1992 Horizon Award—given to the new artist showing the most career growth that year—to Suzy Bogguss, but won Vocal Duo of the Year. In the next dozen years, they'd only lose that title one time—in 2000, when Kentucky's Montgomery Gentry slipped in.

For the next several years, these four Oklahoma-linked acts—Brooks, Gill, McEntire and Brooks & Dunn—would dominate the charts and the awards shows, with Brooks not only becoming the biggest thing in country music, but the top pop-music act of the entire decade. For three years running, 1993 through 1995, these artists made up four-fifths of the top candidates for the CMA's Entertainer of the Year Award, with Alan Jackson the sole finalist with no Sooner State ties. (He finally won in '95, after Gill had taken the first two back to back).

Meanwhile, the other major country-music organization sponsoring an awards show, the West Coast-oriented Academy of Country Music, also recognized the dominance of these Oklahoma performers. From 1990 through 1998, either Brooks (with six awards), Brooks & Dunn (two awards) or McEntire (one award) was named the ACM's Entertainer of the Year.

What began this unprecedented run is harder to pin down than the other Oklahoma-fueled national musical movements in this book. Part of it may have been simply coincidence, with all these supremely talented Okies landing in Nashville within a few years of one another and rising to the top at roughly the same time. Some of it, as we'll see, had to do with Tim DuBois and his work in the record industry. And some may simply involve the old saw about how success breeds success, and once Oklahoma's Brooks showed the world what could come out of the state, Nashville went looking for more.

Before Garth—and Vince, and Brooks & Dunn—however, there was Reba. And for several years in the mid-'80s, she was the standard-bearer for Oklahoma music in Nashville.

I was at the National Finals Rodeo all last week, and I'd stand behind the bucking chutes. People'd drop programs down to me for autographs, and we'd visit. I keep remembering that I've waited seven years for people to even ask for my autograph.

—*Reba McEntire, 1983*

With the release of the film of the same name in 1980, the Urban Cowboy phenomenon produced a fresh run on western-wear stores and country dancehalls by people who'd been formerly uninterested. It also marked the rise of a more pop-oriented style of country music, as artists and producers rushed to meet the new influx of consumers who'd discovered Nashville

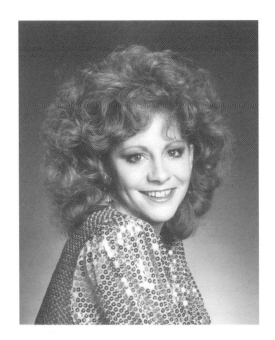

Reba McEntire

and the joys of two-steppin'. The Urban Cowboy movement also seemed to be the catalyst for one of those periodic times when women rise to the top on country-music radio playlists.

Certainly, Oklahoma made more than its share of contributions to that trend. Although she is better known these days as a songwriter—she penned Alabama's No. 1 hit, "I Want to Know You Before We Make Love," among many others—Bartlesville's Becky Hobbs put several songs on the charts in the '80s, including 1983's "Let's Get Over Them Together," a Top 10 duet with Moe Bandy. That same year, Tulsa's Gus Hardin, a club veteran whose achy, soulful vocals had much more to do with the Tulsa Sound than the Nashville sound, was named Top New Female Vocalist by the Academy of Country Music—largely on the strength of her first major-label single, a hit called "After the Last Goodbye."

Then there was Broken Bow's Gail Davies, an almost criminally underrated singer, songwriter, and producer, who blazed a trail for the women who followed her by insisting on doing things the way she felt they should be done. A free-spirited artist with a feminist bent, she produced many of her biggest hits in a time when it was unusual for a woman to take that sort of control in Nashville. Such early- to mid-'80s hits as "Round the Clock Lovin'," "It's A Lovely, Lovely World" and the beautifully nostalgic "Grandma's Song" remain as testaments to her skill and vision as an artist.

Of course, there were male Okies making noise on the charts during this period, too, the most notable being Checotah native Mel McDaniel, whose good-ol'-boy numbers like "Big Ole Brew," "Louisiana Saturday Night" and the No. 1 "Baby's Got Her Blue Jeans On" made him a reliable hitmaker throughout most of the '80s.

But for all of that, it was Reba McEntire who'd become the Queen of Country Music, a title several have worn, but no two at the same time. Her reign began in the mid-'80s and continued throughout most of the '90s. In the new millennium she was still capable of recording a hit, even as she pursued her own TV sitcom,

Reba, and other acting opportunities.

With a father and grandfather who were champion steer ropers, it's logical that McEntire would get some of her first audience exposure at rodeo events. Growing up on a ranch outside of Chockie, a tiny town with a double-digit population, she attended high school in nearby Kiowa, where she and her brother, Pake (who'd later, as a solo act, put a few singles on the country charts, notably the Top 20 hit "Every Night"), and sister Susie (later, as Susie Luchsinger, a well-known contemporary Christian singer), performed at rodeos and other community events as the Singing McEntires.

McEntire's first big break as a solo performer was also rodeo-related. With the help of a couple of famous rodeo figures, Ken Lance and announcer and Oklahoma Senator Clem McSpadden, nineteen-year-old Reba got the high-profile assignment to sing the National Anthem at the 1974 National Finals Rodeo in Oklahoma City. Texan Red Steagall—a western-swing and cowboy music star who was enjoying some success as a country-radio artist—was one of the luminaries present.

Ray Bingham, Steagall's manager—and, for a time, Reba's booking agent—recently recalled how that performance sparked her career.

Ken Lance had the Ken Lance Sports Arena in Ada, Oklahoma, and he always had the Singing McEntires at his rodeo dances. So he'd arranged for her to sing the National Anthem at Oklahoma City.

Justin Boot Company always had a suite in a hotel across the street from where the rodeo was held, and the musicians like Red, and Moe Bandy, all the performers, would go over there and have guitar pulls, you know. Well, after the rodeo, Clem McSpadden and Ken Lance took Reba over and introduced her to Red Steagall.

Reba's mother, Jackie, asked Red, "Would it be possible for you to help my kids?"

Red said, "Let me think about it."

He called Jackie real soon after that and he said, "I'm not sure if I can help the whole family, but I think I might be able to do something for Reba."

Red took her to Nashville, to Mercury Records, and they did a demo and got her a deal. He did that because he just thought she had the potential to be what she turned out to be.

That potential, however, didn't immediately translate into chart success. In fact, her first Top 10 country record didn't come until 1980's "(You Lift Me Up) to Heaven."

In her half-decade as a major-label artist before that, she'd only made the Top 20 of the national country charts a couple of times, once in 1977 with a cover of the Patsy Cline evergreen "Sweet Dreams," the other the next year as half of a duet with Mercury labelmate Jacky Ward on one called "Three Sheets in the Wind."

Once "(You Lift Me Up) to Heaven" broke the barrier, though, it wasn't long before she was hitting the upper reaches of the charts with impressive regularity. Her first No. 1 came with the wry "Can't Even Get the Blues" in 1983, the year that saw her pick up her first two CMA nominations (for the Horizon Award and Female Vocalist of the Year). That was also the year she moved from Mercury/Polygram, which had released her first five albums, to the giant MCA.

"We changed on October 19, when it was time for us to renew our contract on Mercury," McEntire said in a late 1983 interview. "We all talked about it. You know, you stay with one company too long, you get to be like wallpaper. MCA's got people like Barbara [Mandrell] and Loretta [Lynn]—superstars—and we thought they might be able to use someone who was kind of on the way up."

It wouldn't be long before her own name would be included in that august company. With MCA, McEntire reeled off a long string of hit records, many of them going all the way to No. 1. On the strength of those singles—including the likes of "How Blue," "Somebody Should Leave," and "Whoever's in New England"—she became the CMA's Female Vocalist of the Year from '84 through '87, picking up a 1986 Entertainer of the Year Award as well.

To some, McEntire's down-home, aw-shucks persona and Oklahoma-cowgirl accent masked the fact that she was an ambitious and shrewd artist who gradually took more and more control of her own career. She had definite ideas about what she wanted to do and where she wanted to go with her music, and one of the things she began doing was recording songs specifically for women, an audience segment traditionally seen as cool to female artists. For her, however, it

"SHE HAD DEFINITE IDEAS ABOUT WHAT SHE WANTED TO DO AND WHERE SHE WANTED TO GO WITH HER MUSIC, AND ONE OF THE THINGS SHE BEGAN DOING WAS RECORDING SONGS SPECIFICALLY FOR WOMEN, AN AUDIENCE SEGMENT TRADITIONALLY SEEN AS COOL TO FEMALE ARTISTS."

worked. In a 1986 interview, she noted that her brother Pake's wife, who ran Reba's fan club at the time, "says that we've been getting so many more women to join lately."

I've seen it at the autograph table, too. Women don't generally like to listen to or watch other female singers because maybe their husbands or boyfriends are watching, but in my show, I dedicate one song to men and three to women.

Something [on her then-current album, Whoever's in New England] like "I've Seen Better Days" appeals to women now, because some women are losing custody of their kids. That didn't happen 10 years ago. And a song like "One Thin Dime" just kinda says, "Hey, I'm here," and that appeals to women. There's a different attitude. Women are tougher now.

McEntire showed a little toughness herself after the release of 1988's *Reba*, a pop-flavored album that included remakes of the '50s pop hit "Sunday Kind of Love" and Aretha Franklin's signature soul song, "Respect." In an interview that same year, she acknowledged that her recording of those pop numbers shook up some of her fans.

"When those two songs came out, some people were offended. They said, 'Well, Reba's leaving country music.' And I said, 'Really? Come *on*. Listen to the way I *talk*,'" she said, laughing.

People like familiarity, and when someone steps out of that it's a shock to them. But I can't do the same thing over and over again. It limits my growth. It gets stale. And when that happens I get bored. I like to do new things, so people'll say, "Well, what's she gonna do next?"

What's good about being in the country-music field is that the spectrum is so broad. On one end, you've got traditional going into bluegrass, and on the other end it's almost pop. Country music gives you the greatest freedom of all.

"Sunday Kind of Love" went on to become a Top Five country hit, while the Otis Redding-penned "Respect," while never a single, was soon a staple of her increasingly elaborate stage shows. McEntire continued to explore her musical and theatrical boundaries throughout the '90s and into the new millennium, her career surviving the loss of most of her touring band in a 1991 plane crash. Coincidentally, that was the same year that her duet with an up-and-coming Oklahoma act on her label, MCA, became one of the few unabashed western-swing songs to make the country-music Top 10 in the modern hit-radio era. Called "Oklahoma Swing," it would turn out to be a pivotal recording in the career of a young guitarist, songwriter and singer named Vince Gill.

I was famous because I mooned the crowd.

— *Vince Gill*

With an appealingly easygoing personality to go with blazing guitar chops, a pure and emotive tenor voice, and impressive songwriting skills, Norman native Vince Gill was the complete package—a fact not lost on the Nashville establishment. Gill not only hosted the televised Country Music Association Awards for more than a decade, he also

Vince Gill

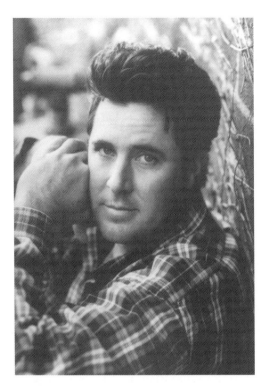

received many of those awards. The self-effacing and immensely talented Okie became the face of country music in the 1990s, a telegenic performer who never failed to emit good vibes.

Like fellow Oklahoman Reba McEntire, Gill's solo career sputtered along at a slow burn for several years before finally igniting. Unlike McEntire, however, well before his ascendancy to solo-act stardom, he worked as a member of several different bands, singing and playing and writing songs. Sometimes, acts who come up in that manner take a little longer to develop, whether because of an aversion to stepping into the spotlight and away from the rest of the band, both symbolically and literally, or because making the music is more important than becoming a star. Because of his days as a guitar-playing member of a group instead of a front-man vocalist, Gill has antecedents in such country stars as Steve Wariner and Ricky Skaggs, crackerjack instrumentalists, vocalists, and writers who spent a lot of time as boys in the band before going on to out-front fame.

In a 1990 interview, Gill remembered the time with his first band, an Oklahoma City-based progressive-bluegrass outfit called Mountain Smoke, as "the most fun I ever had playing music."

What an amazing set of personalities. There was a college student, a sprinkler installer, a music professor, two bankers and me. It was so much fun. I was 17, and hanging out with these men—all grown up, with families, and crazy as a bunch of loons. I had a lot of firsts the year I was with 'em, if you know what I mean.

One of those firsts—and, presumably, a last—came in a mid-'70s show at Oklahoma City's Myriad Convention Center. It's a performance that has become a part of Oklahoma music legend, not only because of Gill's audacious exit strategy, but because someone actually thought pairing a bluegrass band and the then-hugely popular rock group KISS would be a swell idea.

Apparently, the scheduled opening act had to

cancel at the last minute, so the promoters called Mountain Smoke to do the gig. "We were pretty well-known around the area then," explained Gill, "and they used us a lot."

This time, though, it didn't work. The KISS audience was not in the mood to see a bunch of bluegrass jakes open the show for their painted-face rock heroes. Gill remembered how the group nonetheless tried gamely to go on.

"We played as much as we could, until we realized our lives were in danger. They were throwing beer cans at us. Everybody was booing. I'd never heard 5,000 people booing all at once before. One of the guys got scared, and I told him, "They can't hurt you with beer cans. They're empty."

"WE PLAYED AS MUCH AS WE COULD, UNTIL WE REALIZED OUR LIVES WERE IN DANGER. THEY WERE THROWING BEER CANS AT US. EVERYBODY WAS BOOING. I'D NEVER HEARD 5,000 PEOPLE BOOING ALL AT ONCE BEFORE. ONE OF THE GUYS GOT SCARED, AND I TOLD HIM, "THEY CAN'T HURT YOU WITH BEER CANS. THEY'RE EMPTY."

So the band members finally gave up and retreated from the stage, but not before young Gill turned his backside to the crowd for a final, defiant, gesture.

Really, it was pretty funny. The best part about it was the guy who wrote the review for the paper the next day. He said, "It was amazing that Mountain Smoke took it as long as they did. And after they'd had enough, Vince Gill showed the crowd what part of his anatomy they could kiss."

"When I did it," he added, laughing, "the police gave me a standing ovation."

Gill recalled that incident in an interview in January 1990 that was published prior to his playing the Tulsa City Limits dancehall, where a group, much to his amusement, unfurled a giant banner that read: *Vince—Sing 'Moon River'*.

By that time, Gill's Mountain Smoke days were long behind him. After his high school graduation, he'd traveled to Kentucky, where he played with the groups Bluegrass Alliance and Boone Creek, a Ricky Skaggs outfit. A year or so later, he was in Los Angeles, playing with former University of Oklahoma student (and current Guthrie resident) Byron Berline in a group called Sundance.

Prior to going solo, Gill had also spent several years in the pioneering country-rock band Pure Prairie League, singing lead on the smooth pop-country hit "Let Me Love You Tonight" and writing another of the band's hits, the rocking "I'm Almost Ready" (both from 1980). And before the late '80s, when MCA took a chance on him as a solo artist, he'd also been a member of Rodney Crowell's band the Cherry Bombs and worked steadily as a Nashville session player and singer. During those Nashville years, he'd also cut three solo albums that yielded a few decent country hits—notably 1985's "Oklahoma Borderline." His solo career, however, continued to simmer without ever quite coming to a boil.

All of that changed with the 1989 disc *When I Call Your Name*, which included the "Oklahoma Swing" duet with McEntire. Given Gill and McEntire's Oklahoma roots, it's fitting that his breakthrough song was an example of the best-known musical style to come out of the state. Western swing is a musician's music, too, which makes it doubly appropriate for Gill's entrée to the next level.

However, "Oklahoma Swing" was an unlikely vehicle for anyone's stardom. By the time the song came out, western swing had long been considered "niche" music, like bluegrass, by the Nashville establishment, and even huge stars who loved to work in that form, like Texan George Strait, seldom saw their swing tunes hit the very top of the chart. In an interview conducted in September 1990, after "Oklahoma Swing" had completed its run, Gill offered some thoughts about the song, hit-country radio, and western swing in general.

It's so funny about radio. Swing is really a serious early form of country music, but a lot of stations wouldn't play our record because it was western swing. It went to No. 4, which meant that the people who played it played it a lot, but some stations wouldn't touch it. They wouldn't touch any western swing at all.

By the time of that interview, however, Gill didn't have to worry much about the resistance in some quarters to "Oklahoma Swing." His follow-up single, the title track from *When I Call Your Name*, had just become one of the biggest songs of the year. With backing vocals by country star Patty Loveless, it had, as Gill noted at the time, "all the elements of real hard-core country music—and, like my friend [the songwriter] Max Barnes says, it's sadder than a one-car funeral.

"To be around as long as I've been," he added, "and then have this major hit—it was a major, major blessing."

"When I Call Your Name," written by Gill and fellow Oklahoman Tim Dubois, was indeed a huge blessing. It would become the CMA's Single and Song of the Year for 1990, and it would also win Gill a Grammy for Best Country Vocal Performance by a Male. The album of the same name would ultimately go platinum, signifying sales of more than a million copies.

But it was also the beginning of a long run as a country superstar for the Norman native, leading to more platinum albums and major hit singles, big-arena concerts and increased television exposure.

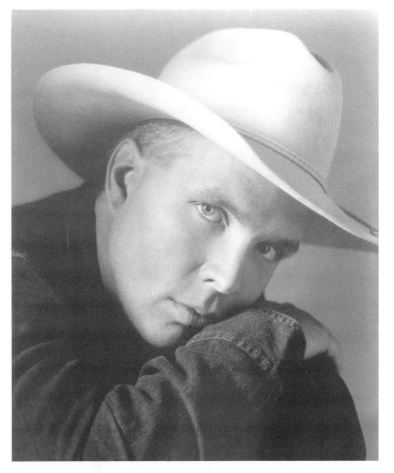

Garth Brooks

Often, the concerts and the television exposure went hand in hand. In 1993, for instance, Gill came into Tulsa—with guests Amy Grant (later to become his wife), Chet Atkins, and Michael McDonald—to do a Christmas concert with the Tulsa Philharmonic Orchestra that was broadcast as a special on the Nashville Network.

In an interview prior to the taping, Gill was asked how he felt about a newspaper writer referring to him as the Perry Como of the '90s. (Later, in 1997, the Kraft company would sponsor Gill's national tour, just as it had sponsored laid-back crooner Como's popular TV shows in the '50s and '60s.) Gill laughed when he answered, "I don't mind that a bit."

It's just the way I am. I can't jump around on stage and do things that aren't natural. A musician's got to be comfortable to play, and I want to be comfortable. I'd wear tennis shoes if they'd let me, but I don't get to do that very often. Besides, Perry Como was cool.

While Gill was, and remains, a cool presence on stage, letting his playing and singing carry the show, another Oklahoma artist who came along in the late '80s couldn't have been more different as a live performer. His wild and frenetic stage shows became one of the reasons he catapulted not only to country music stardom, but well beyond. Garth Brooks, quite simply, became the top pop-music figure of the '90s.

On the surface, there's no great secret to Garth's fame. He is a driven man. Everything he has accomplished he wanted badly. He worked hard. I've never known anyone in any walk of life who was so completely hell-bent on making it to the top. That's why few who know him were surprised Garth entered the spotlight. But when his fame spilled over into the realm of cultural phenomenon, everyone—including Garth—dropped their jaws in disbelief.

— from *Garth Brooks: The Road Out of Santa Fe* by *Matt O'Meilia*

(University of Oklahoma Press, 1997)

There's a saying we live by that says you can't please everybody all the time. But until you've tried, I don't think it's fair to say that.

—*Garth Brooks, 1995*

While it may be a little too pat to define decades of the rock 'n' roll era by individual artists, lots of people do it. The '50s is Elvis' decade, so they say, while the '60s belong to the Beatles, the '70s to Elton John, and the '80s to Michael Jackson.

If you extend that notion to the '90s, there's really only one artist who sums up the closing decade of the 20th Century. Troyal Garth Brooks, a Tulsa native who grew up in Yukon and attended college at Oklahoma State University in Stillwater, was the biggest-selling recording act of the '90s, celebrating astounding album sales of 100 million with a Nashville party in October of 2000. No other solo artist had ever sold that many records, and only the Beatles had sold more—but they hadn't done it in a decade, as Garth had. At this writing, he's *still* selling CDs by the millions, even though he announced his retirement from active participation in the music business in November, 2000, a month or so after the soiree celebrating his unprecedented album-selling achievements. He's the biggest-selling single artist in popular-music history, and even if he stopped selling records tomorrow, his incredible total isn't likely to be topped anytime soon.

For a decade-long stretch, Brooks also routinely sold out stadiums in America and across the world, and, according to *The Encyclopedia of Country Music* (Oxford University Press, 1998), drew an astounding quarter of a million people to his 1997 show in New York City's Central Park. If, as the singer-songwriter Kathy Mattea has said, country music became the genre that talks about being a grownup in the United States, then Brooks was the man most responsible for that change, breaking country music into the mainstream by masterfully blending elements of rock, folk, and pop into his country records and stage performances. Not a crossover artist in the accepted sense of the term—his biggest hit

"HE'S THE BIGGEST-SELLING SINGLE ARTIST IN POPULAR-MUSIC HISTORY, AND EVEN IF HE STOPPED SELLING RECORDS TOMORROW, HIS INCREDIBLE TOTAL ISN'T LIKELY TO BE TOPPED ANYTIME SOON."

on the pop charts was 1999's Top Five "Lost in You," done when he was trying out his alter ego of Chris Gaines, a fabricated rock 'n' roll star—he brought country music out of the honky-tonks and dancehalls of the South, Southwest and West and spread it across the nation, attracting millions of new people to the genre. The *Urban Cowboy* movie made dancing to country music acceptable to a whole new audience; Garth Brooks' music, coming along a decade later, made *listening* to country music acceptable to a much bigger segment of America.

In 1997, Tulsa's Matt O'Meilia wrote an account of his time playing drums with the group Santa Fe, which featured both Brooks and Red Dirt music pioneer Tom Skinner, among others. Published by the University of Oklahoma Press, *Garth Brooks: The Road out of Santa Fe* indicates that Brooks knew exactly what he wanted a long time before his stardom. Author O'Meilia introduced the book with a paragraph that neatly telegraphs his bandmate's intentions.

Driving back from the Bamboo Ballroom in Enid, Oklahoma, one early Sunday morning, Garth and I were musing about fame and fortune. Idle talk, I thought, until Garth blurted out, "I want to be. . .America's Band!" Even through the gloom of the car interior I could see his eyes burning with intensity.

Brooks had come to Stillwater from Yukon, where he'd played football, baseball, basketball, and track. He was enough of an athlete to get a partial scholarship in, of all things, the javelin, and enough of an academic to graduate in December 1984 with an advertising degree. He also had enough country music in his background that a career in it didn't seem so far-fetched—his mother, Colleen Carroll, had recorded for Capitol in the '50s and was a regional headliner for several years. "If I do have any talent," he said in a 1989 interview, "it's from her."

By the time Santa Fe came along, Brooks had already been playing as a single in various Stillwater venues, including a place called Willie's, where he might follow a George Jones tune with a Dan Fogelberg number, and then launch into "Beth" by KISS or another rock-band ballad. In publicity material from the early '90s, he lists all those acts as influences, and that fact goes a long way toward explaining how, even then, he was blending music from a lot of different genres into his work, paving the way for a new sound that would end up captivating much of the country.

By 1986, he'd also taken his first run at Nashville, a discouraging and unsuccessful experience. However, he found new hope with Santa Fe, a band that mixed music from the likes of Bob Seger, Lynyrd Skynyrd and James Taylor with their country covers. The approach fit perfectly with Brooks' eclecticism, and by 1988, he was back in Music City, this time with the rest of the group along for the ride. In the 1989 interview, he noted that the band members gave themselves six months to make it, but Santa Fe ended up falling apart before that time expired.

You stick five guys, two wives, a kid and a dog and cat in one house, and try and see how you deal with the unknown. I'm telling you, it's scarier than hell. On top of that, we all had our own different ways of dealing with things, and as a result, everything just kind of fell apart. There were some hard feelings, but not as many as you might think. We're still all interested in what the other ones are doing. We still speak to each other. But it was real scary. Nobody knew what was going on.

The day after the prearranged six-month period was up, Brooks signed a songwriting contract with a Nashville publishing house, where he met a Nashville music figure named Bob Doyle. Doyle was interested in forming a management company, and so was his associate Pam Lewis.

They thought the new kid in town might be a nice way to start out, so they joined forces and began pushing Garth. "A couple of months later," he recalled, "I had a record deal." Interestingly enough, it was with Capitol Records, his mother's former label.

Brooks' first single release, "Much Too Young (To Feel This Damn Old)," a rodeo-rider lament that gave a nod to fellow artist Chris LeDoux, soared into the country-music Top 10, and Brooks assembled a six-man band and hit the road. He called the group Stillwater, after the town where his music got going, and included an old OSU roommate in the outfit. Oklahoma City native Ty England would tour as a guitarist and backup vocalist with Brooks for several years, and then leave the group—with Garth's blessings—to begin a solo career. His first major-label single, 1995's "Should've Asked Her Faster," remains his biggest hit as a solo act, although he has continued to work live shows and record.

From the beginning, Brooks and Stillwater gave audiences a country-music show that simply didn't look like any of the rest in the genre. While other country acts, notably LeDoux, had been using pyrotechnics and other whizzy accouterments for a few years, Brooks and his sidemen on stage gave off a frenetic aura not seen since the golden days of the rock 'n' rolling Paul Revere and the Raiders. The whooping, shouting, and mugging weren't the only things that riveted attention on the stage, though. Even that early, Brooks showed himself to be a masterful manipulator of emotion, delivering his homegrown lyrics with sincerity and power. A Brooks show made for an emotional roller-coaster ride, and it only got better as he went along.

By early 1990, he'd already logged three very

different hits—"Much Too Young (To Feel This Damn Old)," the uncompromisingly sentimental ballad "If Tomorrow Never Comes," and a raucous honky-tonker called "Not Counting You." He'd co-written all three of the songs, and in an interview at the time, he invoked the name of another singer-songwriter, who also happened to be one of his old bandmates. "For me," Garth said, "the music is the thing. Tom Skinner said it best when we had the group Santa Fe: If you don't have original music, it's like having a sandwich with no meat in it.

"What I want to do," he added, "is for people to hear each new song of mine and say, 'What the hell was *that*?' And then, when they find out it's me, say, 'Hey, that's completely different from the last thing he did.'"

Later that same year, Brooks won the first of his 11 (at this writing) Country Music Association Awards, nabbing the Horizon Award and Music Video of the Year honors. The latter was for his hit "The Dance," a song about risking pain in order to live fully, and the video—featuring images of murdered historical figures like Martin Luther King and John F. Kennedy—gave some of the first indications that Brooks wasn't afraid of making powerful and even controversial statements with his work.

Four years later, he was riding high as not only the biggest thing in country music, but also as the most successful and influential pop star of the decade. His first greatest-hits collection—an 18-cut, two-CD package—had just come out, and four of his hit numbers weren't even on it. "When I look at this album," he said at the time, "I see a lot of inspiration. I see a lot of . . . I don't know if 'passion' is the word or not."

I don't know if other people are like this, but sometimes I just enjoy being upset, going through trials, like in "Rodeo" and "The Thunder Rolls." I enjoy postcards from the past, like "Last Summer." If there's a common thread that runs through all of this, it's that I, Garth Brooks, believe what all these songs are saying.

Tellingly, his favorite song on the collection was "The Dance," that Tony Arata composition about taking chances regardless of the possible consequences. Anyone wanting to understand Brooks and his approach to his music has to understand that the idea of trying new things was essential, as was acting on emotions—both of which are addressed in "The Dance."

Also, as a man with an advertising degree, he knew well one of the basic principles of marketing: Every so often, you have to change the look of a successful product, or it'll fade from public interest. Remember that element of Brooks' schooling, and you'll get a good idea of why he not only did a whole disc in the late '90s as a fictional pop star

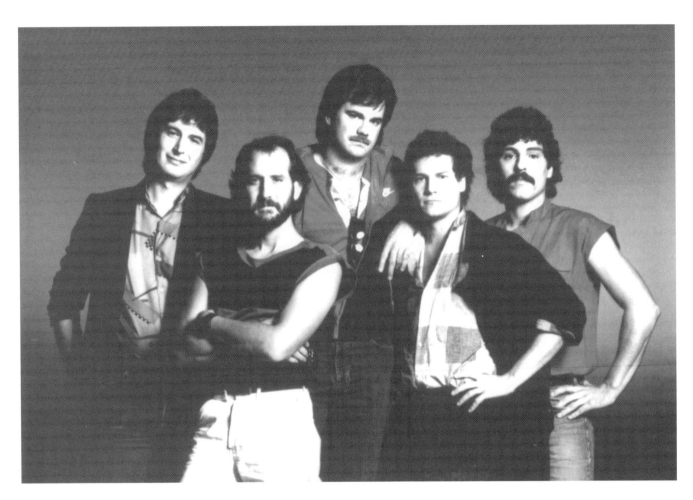

Restless Heart

named Chris Gaines, but virtually starved himself to get the sunken-cheeked rock-star appearance he has on the CD's packaging. It baffled a lot of his audience, but it was—just like his spring-training appearances with major-league teams—an at-bat he felt he needed to take.

Another thing to consider about Brooks is his genuine humility. He may have crossed over all kinds of boundaries with his addition of other elements to country music, but he surely embodied one of the genre's classic traditions. From the very earliest days of hillbilly music, its practitioners took great pains to present themselves as just plain folks, not really any different—except maybe luckier—than the people paying to see them perform. Putting on airs back then, copping an attitude, especially publicly, was a sure way to alienate a country audience. While that idea began to look increasingly quaint as the modern country era rolled on, Brooks continued to embody it in its purest form. In the interview about his first greatest-hit disc, for instance, he said, "I've always wanted to be one of the people. I've wanted to speak for the people. I don't want to dictate. I don't want to rule. I just want to be a voice."

Certainly, that attitude could be put on in front of audiences and taken off backstage, like one of those brightly decorated jackets favored by country singers of a certain era. But with Brooks, it appeared genuine. For an international superstar with insane demands on his time and attention, he handled being the biggest pop star in the world about as humbly as it could be handled. Tim Miller, the Chickasha-born director of Brooks' "We Shall Be Free" video—which was, in its visualization of the song's plea for tolerance for all people, a somewhat controversial work—recalled in 1994 how Brooks pitched in to get the video done in time for an airing as part of the January Super Bowl telecast.

I've worked with everyone from Tom Brokaw to Bill Cosby, and Garth is the warmest, most loving, man I've ever met at that level of celebrity. He's a very gracious man. He was there to help us unload the trucks. He was there to run and get food. He was, really, one of the guys.

You know, people say I have the reputation of giving an act from Oklahoma 25 extra points—and I probably do. There's something special about Oklahoma. I've been asked about this before, and I think it's more than just being prejudiced toward people from Oklahoma. There really is something there, something better.

—*Tim DuBois,*
record-company executive and native Oklahoman, 1993

To cover the career of the fourth huge Oklahoma-connected country star to burst out in the early '90s, it's necessary to go back more than a decade to see what some other Oklahoma country-music figures were up to at the time. Grove's Tim DuBois, for instance, had graduated from Oklahoma State University a decade and a half before Garth Brooks, earning bachelor's and master's degrees in accounting. In the late '70s and early '80s, he'd been a professor of accounting at three different Nashville colleges. But the reason he's germane to this discussion was that at the same time, he was quietly becoming a major country-music songwriter, writing or co-writing such hits as Alabama's "Love in the First Degree," Jerry Reed's "She Got the Gold Mine (I Got the Shaft)," and Razzy Bailey's "Midnight Hauler," among many others.

Clinton's Scott Hendricks, meanwhile, had been a classmate, friend, and musical cohort of Dubois at OSU, as had guitarist-vocalist Greg Jennings, who hailed from Nicoma Park. By the late '70s, all three were working in Nashville. Altus' Paul Gregg, a singer and bassist, joined them in '78, and a few years later, so did keyboardist-vocalist David Innis of Bartlesville.

For a few years, the group worked on a lot of songwriter demos, demonstration recordings used to pitch songs to artists. Then, in 1983, DuBois and Hendricks put Jennings, Gregg and Innes together with two non-Okies—drummer-vocalist John Dittrich and singer Larry Stewart—and came up with the band Restless Heart, a smooth country-rock group whose layered harmonies immediately invited comparison to the West Coast supergroup the Eagles. But while the Eagles had found most of their success on the pop rather than the country charts, Restless Heart would make its biggest impression at hit-country radio, only occasionally crossing over onto the pop charts (most successfully with the No. 1 country hit "I'll Still be Loving You" in 1987) and into the adult-contemporary market.

With DuBois and Hendricks as the production and engineering team, and DuBois contributing songs, Restless Heart charged out of the gate with a Top 30 country hit in 1985, "Let the Heartache Ride." Soon, the group was a major hitmaker for RCA, producing such late-'80s chart-toppers as "Wheels," "Bluest Eyes in Texas" and "That Rock

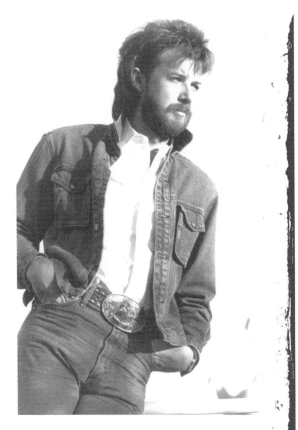

Ronnie Dunn

Won't Roll." In the '90s, Restless Heart underwent several personnel changes and even disbanded for a time, although at the writing the original members of the band are back together, touring and recording.

Meanwhile, both Hendricks and DuBois became major Music City players. Hendricks began producing acts like Alan Jackson, Lee Roy Parnell (a Texan who spent time as a Tulsa resident), Faith Hill, Steve Wariner and Trace Atkins, while DuBois—who didn't quit his day job as a college teacher until the fall of '85—was

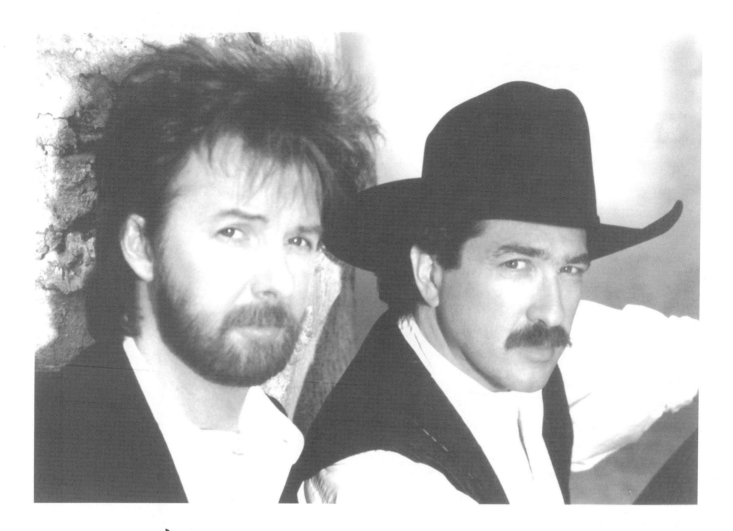

Brooks & Dunn

tabbed by the giant Arista Records to head its new Nashville offices. That was in 1989.

A year earlier, a lanky cat named Ronnie Dunn had parlayed his blow-you-away honky-tonk voice into a first-place finish in the 1988 national Marlboro Country Music Talent Roundup, besting more than 3,800 other contestants from across the country. He had help from a crackerjack band, put together by Tulsa Sound drummer Jamie Oldaker and featuring four musicians—including Oldaker himself—who would later record with singer-songwriter-guitarist Steve Ripley as the Tractors, getting a platinum album in the process.

"What happened was that I went into a QuikTrip and was going to buy something, and I saw the little pamphlets they [Marlboro] had out about the contest," recalled Oldaker in a 1988 conversation. "I read one of 'em, and I said, 'That seems easy enough.' We were having some trouble getting people to see Ronnie in Tulsa, so we decided to do it this way and see what happened."

Dunn, a Texas transplant who could write as well as sing, had been working around Tulsa for well over a decade. After beating the other national finalists on the stage of Nashville's Bullpen Lounge, he was awarded $30,000 and a 40-hour session in a Nashville studio with producer Barry Beckett.

Dunn had been to Music City before. In fact, he'd been there in '84 as a recording artist for the Tulsa-based Churchill Records, where he and famed circus clown Emmett Kelly, Jr.—in a promotion dreamed up by Jim Halsey—had spent a day promoting Dunn's single "She Put the Sad in All His Songs" up and down Music Row.

Some four years later, when Dunn headed into the studio with Beckett, Scott Hendricks was there as well. It's important to note that Dunn recorded his composition "Boot Scootin' Boogie," later to be a huge hit, with those two producers. Just as important, though, is Hendricks' presence at the session. He'd later introduce Dunn to Tim DuBois, thereby setting into motion the events that made Dunn half of the most successful country-music duo of all time.

[Tim DuBois] said, "You're not in Tennessee, and you have to be present to win."

—*Ronnie Dunn, 1991*

In the summer of 1990, Ronnie Dunn was at the top of the country-music scene in Tulsa, but, despite a couple of good tries and the Marlboro win, he hadn't quite been able to make the jump to national stardom. That all began to change with a phone call from Tim DuBois at Arista Nashville. DuBois had signed the veteran Texas-based western-swing band Asleep at the Wheel (which, over the years, has featured a number of Oklahoma players) to the label, and he wanted the group to cut Dunn's "Boot Scootin' Boogie." As it turned out, DuBois was also planning a trip to Grove to visit his parents, and he and Dunn made arrangements to meet for lunch during DuBois' visit.

They met, and DuBois told Dunn that the only thing keeping him out of the country-music mainstream was his location. "And he told me," recalled Dunn in 1991, "that if I wanted to move to Nashville, he'd help me out."

DuBois was as good as his word. After Dunn hit town and rented a house, DuBois helped him get a job as a songwriter with Tree, the largest music publisher in Nashville. Then, one day, DuBois dropped by to take Dunn to lunch. The producer and label head had an ulterior motive, as Dunn recalled.

He told me there was a guy he wanted me to write with, and it turned out to be Kix Brooks. We all had lunch together, and Tim said, "You guys spend some

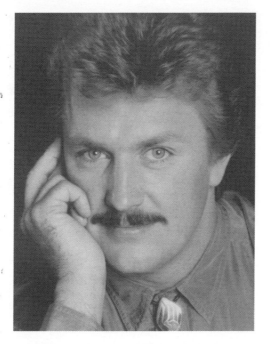

Joe Diffe

time together, hang out together, write some songs together. See how it works out."

The first song we wrote together was "Working on My Next Broken Heart," which is going to be our next single. We demoed it for Tim and he said, "Well, that's what I thought. You guys are an act."

We were shocked, because we were both going after solo deals. But Tim said if we wanted a home, we had it at Arista. And it's just been the red carpet ever since. It hasn't even soaked in yet.

Dunn's comments were made in September 1991, when the duo's first single, "Brand New Man," had surprised everyone by charging out of nowhere to reach No. 1 on every national country chart in America. That was the month that Brooks & Dunn's debut album of the same name (with Scott Hendricks as one of the producers) hit the market. It, too, would be a runaway best-seller, yielding several hits and remaining on the country album charts for an amazing five-plus years.

Like Dunn, Louisiana native Brooks had taken some good shots at a solo career, He'd even been on the Capitol Records roster, recording an album for the label in 1989. Also like Dunn, he was a good songwriter—by the time the two met, his writing credits included such hits as John Conlee's "I'm Only in It for the Love" and the Nitty Gritty Dirt Band's "Modern Day Romance." And, in addition to his singing and songwriting skills, Brooks would bring a kinetic presence to the duo's live shows.

"Kix is a pretty outgoing, wild, Louisiana boy," noted Dunn at the time. "I'm a little more reserved, but I'm getting better."

As the act evolved, however, Dunn was the one who stood and sang most of the lead vocals while Brooks was the rowdy half of the two, dancing and strutting and running around, chopping away at his guitar even as he added solid harmonies to the songs. It wasn't long before these opposites were attracting huge audiences. The unanticipated success of their first single, "Brand New Man," had gotten them out on the road in a hurry in 1991, where they'd started playing mostly clubs.

By 1995, they were headlining arenas. (It should be noted that guitarist Danny MacBride, who was in the band Jamie Oldaker put together for Dunn's Marlboro Country Music Roundup appearances, went on the road with Brooks & Dunn.)

Somewhere between the clubs and the arenas came a number that's still considered their signature song. As noted earlier, Dunn had recorded his composition "Boot Scootin' Boogie" in the late '80s as a solo artist, using the studio time he'd won from the Marlboro Country Music Roundup. Asleep at the Wheel had covered it on the 1990 disc "Keepin' Me Up Nights," the venerable group's only disc for Tim DuBois and Arista Nashville. But none of that even began to anticipate the success the tune would have when recorded by Brooks & Dunn. The last single released from the "Brand New Man" album, it not only shot to the top of the charts, but also became the basis for a music video that was still being shown in country nightspots well over a decade later.

Both an observation of the club scene from the stage and a celebration of country dancing—especially line dancing—"Boot Scootin' Boogie" was a staple of Dunn's repertoire well before he joined Brooks. In fact, it had been the only original song he'd performed during the Marlboro Talent Roundup competitions in 1988. So it was only fitting that when it came time to do the video, he brought a crew from Nashville to the Oklahoma nightspot that had helped inspire the tune.

Tulsa City Limits had become the premiere country nightspot in Tulsa in 1986, following the demise of the *Urban Cowboy*-inspired Duke's Country. Dunn had played both venues dozens of times in his pre-stardom days, and had, for a time, been the front man in the Duke's house band. He'd debuted "Boot Scootin' Boogie" during a set at Tulsa City Limits.

"When you're a cover band, doing other people's music, a lot of people won't get up and dance when you do an original," he recalled in a conversation at the club in May 1992, the day of the video shoot. "But they got right up and danced to it."

After it came out as a track on "Brand New Man," Dunn began pushing for "Boot Scootin' Boogie" to be released as a single, but, he said, "At first, they thought it was too rock-oriented, too punchy. They thought it wouldn't sell in the Northeast. But we started playing up there, and we found out that just about every place we played had a boot-scootin' night every week."

The song jump-started the country line-dancing fad that had become popular in the wake of the Urban Cowboy phenomenon, and the Tulsa City Limits-shot video accurately captured for all time the frenetic lines of friends, acquaintances and total strangers whirling and stepping together in synchronized patterns on the packed, smoky floor of a country-music dancehall.

If they'd only contributed "Boot Scootin' Boogie" to the national music scene, Brooks & Dunn would have a secure place in country music history. But, at the dawn of Oklahoma's centennial year, the two are still cutting hits and winning awards. Those awards began in 1992 with their Country Music Association nod for Vocal Duo of the Year, reaching a peak in 1996, when both the CMA and the Academy of Country Music named them Entertainer of the Year. They've also shown a predilection for working with Oklahoma acts, taking Bethel Acres' Wade Hayes ("Old Enough to Know Better," "Don't Stop") along as their opening act in 1995, and pairing up with Reba McEntire for a blockbuster late '90s tour.

Yet, even in the middle of their huge mid-'90s run, Ronnie Dunn admitted that he was "so neurotic" about his career that it made his wife crazy. "I'll come in and I'll be moping around the house, worrying about the new album, and she'll say, 'Slow down. Relax. You've got enough money now.'

"But for me," he added, "it's like having to get up for playing in the Super Bowl every day, against a real good team."

While the quartet of Brooks, Gill, McEntire and Dunn were the most visible artists during the Okie siege of Nashville in the early '90s, there were other important Oklahoma acts as well. As far as hitmaking goes, the next tier of stars would have to begin with singer-songwriter Joe Diffie, a Tulsa native who lived in various Oklahoma towns during his youth and worked at a foundry in Duncan as an adult—"making valve castings, everything from plumber's elbows to 300-lb. valves," he recalled in a 1991 interview. While in Duncan he sang in a gospel group, worked in a bluegrass act called Special Edition, and put together his own recording studio.

Then, in 1986, events transpired that propelled Diffie to Nashville.

"They closed the foundry down during the big oil bust," he explained. "I got divorced and I just figured I'd kick myself the rest of my life if I didn't go down there and try it."

Working at the Nashville Gibson guitar factory by day, Diffie honed his songwriting and singing skills by night, gradually becoming one of the most sought-after demo singers in town. Once, he recalled, he sang on 13 demos in one day.

Diffie's first hit came in 1990—the year he quit working at Gibson—with the heartfelt ballad "Home." The Epic Records release was his first major-label single, and it made it to the top of the national country charts. A nice run of big radio songs followed, including another poignant ballad, "Ships That Don't Come In." However, as his career rolled on, Diffie became better known for honky-tonk rockers like "Prop Me Up Beside the Jukebox (If I Die)," "If the Devil Danced (In Empty Pockets)," "John Deere Green," and the smash hit "Pickup Man." He was nominated for the 1992 Male Vocalist of the Year Award by the CMA, losing to fellow Okie Vince Gill.

As one might surmise, the six-man group Little Texas had roots in the Lone Star State, even though the name actually came from an area south of Nashville known for its lawlessness in the '20s and '30s. Two of its members, however, had Oklahoma ties. Guitarist Dwayne O'Brien was an Ada native with a degree in chemistry from East Central Oklahoma State University, while vocalist Tim Rushlow was born at Tinker Air Force Base in Midwest City, where his father, Tom, worked. (Tom Rushlow was also the lead vocalist in the popular R&B-flavored show band, Moby Dick & the Whalers, a regional favorite during the late '60s and early '70s.)

After signing a development deal with Warner Brothers in 1988, Little Texas spent the next two and a half years crisscrossing the country, playing three and four sets a night in clubs, honing their chops as a band. All the work paid off in 1991, when the first Little Texas single, the lush "Some Guys Have All the Love," went Top 10. With rich harmonies and road-tested performance ability to go with their teen-appeal looks, the members of Little Texas charted several more singles in the first half of the '90s, including "Amy's Back in Austin," "My Love," and "God Blessed Texas."

The band's high-water mark came in 1994, when it was nominated for Vocal Group of the Year by both the Academy of Country Music and the Country Music Association. It won the first, but lost the second honor to Diamond Rio.

Little Texas disbanded in 1997, following several personnel changes, but reformed a few years later without Rushlow, who busied himself with a solo career. In 2006, he became affiliated with fellow Oklahoman Toby Keith's record label, Show Dog Nashville, which signed him and his cousin, Doni Gene Harris—a former member of the touring band Lariat—as a duet.

Coming along just a bit after the others was Lawton's Bryan White, who was only 20 when he saw the release of his first major-label album in 1994. A singer-songwriter who was also adept at both guitar and drums—a White concert usually allowed its star several opportunities to thump the skins—he scored No. 1 hits like "Someone Else's Star" and "Rebecca Lynn"; toured with another country-star youngster, LeAnn Rimes; and won the CMA's Horizon Award and the ACM's Best New Male Vocalist honors, both in 1996.

Tulsa native Jeff Carson was a rarity—a performer from Branson, Missouri who became a Nashville recording star. Making the jump from Branson in 1989, Carson worked in Music City for half a decade before getting his record deal. A year later, in 1995, his single "Not on Your Love" hit the top of the charts. Another Top Five hit, "The Car," came out the same year. Carson was touring with the Honky Tonk Tailgate Tour package show in 2001, when the success of his Top 20 country single "Real Life (Never Was the Same Again)" gave his career a renewed boost, and he left the tour and began working solo again.

Another Oklahoma artist who spent some time with the Honky Tonk Tailgate Tour was the aforementioned Wade Hayes, whose father, Don, had seen some success in the Oklahoma area as a country-music singer. Influenced by western swing, honky-tonk, and classic country, the younger Hayes had a nice run of hits in the mid-'90s, and surfaced again in the early part of the 21st Century as half of the duo McHayes, with his Oklahoma friend Mark McClurg, a Claremore native who played fiddle in Alan Jackson's road band. The two had met when Hayes was on the road as Jackson's opening act, and McClurg had later played in the Honky Tonk Tailgate Tour road band behind Hayes.

By the time McHayes came along in 2003, Tim DuBois was heading a new label, Universal South, and he and partner Tony Brown signed McHayes to a deal. Unfortunately, despite the undeniable talent of the duo, Brooks & Dunn-style lightning didn't strike again for DuBois, and McHayes disbanded before its first disc could be officially released.

Like Little Texas, Ricochet was a band forged in the crucible of the national country-nightclub scene, its members coming from hardworking cover bands with names like Singletree and Lariat (which had also featured Tim Rushlow's cousin Doni Harris at one point). Singer and lead guitarist Heath Wright and bassist-vocalist Greg Cook, boyhood friends and musical compadres from Vian, became founding members of Ricochet, which thundered out of the gate in 1996 with a couple of major hits, the ballad "What Do I Know" and the peppy "Daddy's Money." On the strength of that debut, Ricochet earned both Top Vocal Group and Top New Vocal Group honors from the Academy of Country Music.

The band, however, may be best-known for its a cappella rendition of "The Star-Spangled Banner," which it began doing in its stage shows following the April 1995 bombing of the Oklahoma City Federal Building. Ricochet's version of the National Anthem became so popular that the six-man group recorded it—and, surprisingly, hit the national country charts with it as well.

"We're the only country act ever to chart

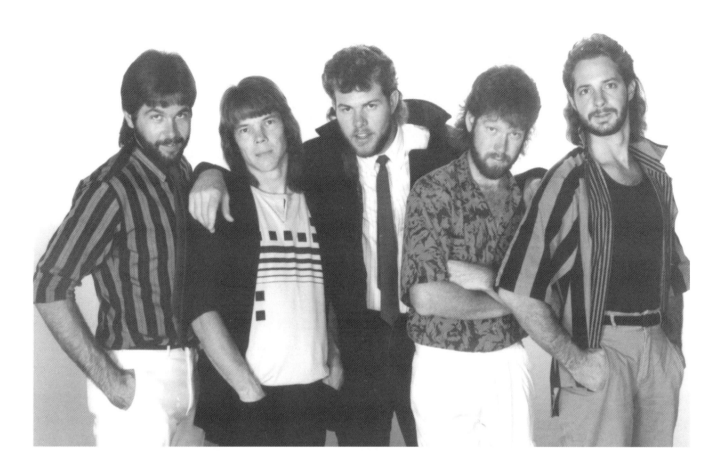

Easy Money
Toby Keith in middle

'The Star-Spangled Banner,'" said Wright with a chuckle during a 1996 interview. "It came out the week 'Daddy's Money' went to No. 1. It was just after the July 4th weekend, so 'The Star-Spangled Banner' had gotten a lot of spins. 'Daddy's Money' was No. 1 on the *Billboard* chart, and 'Star-Spangled Banner' was the Hot Shot Debut. I still have that chart."

These performers—led by the Big Four of Brooks, Gill, McEntire, and Dunn, and reinforced by a couple of others we'll look at shortly—were the reason that Oklahoma artists dominated the hit-country radio charts in the first half-dozen or so years of the '90s, an occurrence that hasn't happened before or since.

What was the reason? In a 1991 interview with the *Tulsa Tribune's* Ellis Widner, Capitol Records Nashville executive Buzz Stone, who'd worked with Reba McEntire at MCA, said, "There's quite

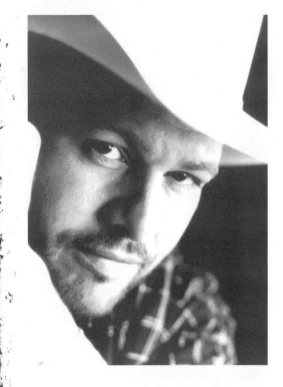

Toby Keith

a talent pool in Oklahoma. Music seems to be a part of the people's lives there, more so than in other states."

In the same story, Tony Brown—Tim DuBois' Universal South partner, who was then an MCA Nashville exec as well as Vince Gill's producer—noted that "Oklahoma and Texas always have been obvious places to look for country talent. Texas always seems to feel it carries the banner, but the Okies are running head-to-head with them."

Neither of those observations, however, explains why the explosion happened when it did. There may not be an explanation beyond the general notions of coincidence and timing; then again, an old baseball axiom might be apt here. The saying is that good hitting is contagious—so, if one or two batters on a team catch fire, many times their teammates will heat up at the plate as well. In the very early '90s, when McEntire had already established herself as a headliner and Brooks was coming on like gangbusters—as were Gill and Brooks & Dunn—their Sooner State counterparts were not only inspired to take a run at stardom themselves, but perhaps treated a little differently by record-company executives simply because of their state of origin. That theory doesn't even take into account producers and label guys like Tim DuBois and Scott Hendricks, transplanted Okies themselves, who undoubtedly gave nascent Oklahoma acts a little extra attention.

We'll also never know the extent of the help that the performers gave each other, in that great Oklahoma tradition of brotherhood and consideration for one another that marked the lives and work of their musical forebears. Some of it is a matter of record: Brooks going back and picking up his old Oklahoma State University pal Ty England, later helping him make the transition to a solo act, and superstar McEntire pairing with Gill—whose career wasn't nearly as far along at hers at that point—to help create the breakthrough Gill single "Oklahoma Swing."

It's also worth noting that, in addition to that western-swing number, Gill and McEntire, as well as Dunn and Brooks, tipped their Stetsons to the music of home-state boy Bob Wills by appearing on tribute discs put together by Texas' Ray Benson and his long-lived swing band Asleep at the Wheel. On the all-star 1993 collection *A Tribute to the Music of Bob Wills and the Texas Playboys,* Garth sang "Deep Water," while Brooks & Dunn did "Corrine, Corrina," and Gill performed "Yearning (Just for You)," all Wills standards. Gill also played guitar on the instrumental "Red Wing," which won him (as well as the great Wills guitarist Eldon Shamblin) a Grammy for Best Country Instrumental Performance.

On Asleep at the Wheel's follow-up disc, 2000's *Ride with Bob*, Gill was back again, playing with a number of other top-flight guitarists—including Wills associate and Oklahoman Tommy Allsup—on the instrumental "Bob's Breakdowns," for which they received another Grammy. Also on that disc, McEntire contributed her vocals to the Wills classic "Right or Wrong."

Some of these acts had connections to the classic Tulsa Sound as well, with the biggest example seen in the makeup of the band that helped Ronnie Dunn win the 1988 Marlboro Country Music Roundup. Many of those players, who'd already been major contributors to the Tulsa Sound of the '70s, would eventually work back in Tulsa with a former Stillwater music figure, record producer and engineer, and Bob Dylan sideman named Steve Ripley. As the Tractors, they'd create a million-plus-selling debut disc for Tim DuBois' Arista Nashville label, which we'll look at in the next chapter.

And finally, a young man from Moore also began to make his mark in country music during this golden age of the Nashville Okies. Toby Keith, however, while knocking out several hits in the early to mid-'90s, would bounce around from record label to record label and never really achieve his huge stardom until the early part of the 21st Century.

A former oilfield worker and minor-league football player (for the Oklahoma City Drillers, a team in the now-defunct United States Football League), Keith paid years of dues in the '80s and early '90s as a member of the hard-touring bar band Easy Money. In a 1993 interview, Keith recalled those tough days of relentlessly hitting the road and taking home "six grand a year with a baby on the way."

By the late '80s, however, the group was doing well enough to switch from a van to a Silver Eagle bus, even though road-weary members were dropping out and being replaced at a rapid pace. By 1992, when Keith signed his solo deal with Mercury

Records, he was the only founding member left.

When Keith's first single, "Should've Been A Cowboy," hit the charts in '93, he was on the road again with a package show called the Mercury Triple Play Tour. The traveling concert featured three new Mercury acts—Keith, Shania Twain and singer-songwriter John Brannen—each getting a half-hour solo spot in front of the same road band. Hardly a stranger to the road, Keith was in the middle of the Mercury tour when he called it "the most tiring thing I've ever done."

With Easy Money, you'd drive to the club and load in on Tuesday night, and then you could sleep all day Wednesday. You played every night through Saturday, but you had the whole week to golf or whatever during the day.

This tour has been, like, three hours of sleep a day for six weeks. We've been averaging [appearances on] three TV stations a day, three or four radio stations, and talking to a couple of newspapers, and sometimes the local country-music magazines, too. And then, we've sometimes had as many as 15 phoners [telephone interviews] on the off days.

Still, he added, he wasn't complaining.

"This is playing hardball with the big boys," he said. "This isn't opening a show, where you go out and do cover stuff and everyone's waiting for the star. This is a once-in-a-lifetime opportunity. Sure, it's a little tiring. But this is why we sing."

It all paid off for Keith, who saw that first single hit the upper reaches of the charts, followed by similar hits like "He Ain't Worth Missing" and "A Little Less Talk and a Lot More Action." A switch to Polydor Records in '94 yielded the likes of "Who's That Man" and "You Ain't Much Fun (Since I Quit Drinkin')."

By 1998, after five albums and a string of hit singles, Keith saw the release of his first greatest-hits package, which went platinum (signifying sales of more than a million copies). For all that reliable hitmaking, however, it still took a couple more label changes and the 1999 disc *How Do You Like Me Now* to catapult him into the rarefied air of country-music superstardom, as he became best-known for the kind of attitude-packed, testosterone-fueled, chip-on-the-shoulder numbers that had made Hank Williams Jr. a huge star in the 1980s. While any number of Keith hits in the early part of the 21st Century (including "How Do You Like Me Now," "I Wanna Talk About Me" and "Who's Your Daddy") make good illustrations, the prime example is 2002's "Courtesy of the Red, White & Blue (the Angry American)," a wildly patriotic, bellicose shake of his fist (and thrust of his boot) at America's enemies.

At this writing, Keith—on the strength of his status as one of the top touring and recording acts in all of pop music—has once again changed record companies, this time establishing his own label, Big Dog Nashville. As mentioned earlier, one of the first acts he signed was fellow Oklahoma native, and former Little Texas member, Tim Rushlow.

7
CHAPTER SEVEN
RED DIRT ROADS

IT'S kind of hard to put into words, but if you ever drive down on the [Mississippi] Delta, you can almost hear that blues sound. Go to New Orleans, and you can almost hear the Dixieland jazz. Go to San Francisco, and you get that psychedelic-music vibe. You hear the Red Dirt sound when you go through Stillwater. It has to do with the spirit of the people. They're Okies, and I think the whole Red Dirt sound is just as important to American musicology as the San Francisco sound or any of the rest. It's distinctly its own thing.
    —Jimmy LaFave, 2002

IT all gets down to whether you're writing for your heart or your pocketbook, and around here, we seem to be writing from the heart.
    —Mike McClure, 2002

The reader who's gotten this far knows that this book is primarily concerned with a couple of things. First, it's about the musical movements that swept out of Oklahoma and through the popular music of the nation and the world over the years, beginning with the influence the Oklahoma City Blue Devils had on the sound of jazz in general and Kansas City jazz in particular. The second is the theory that Oklahoma's music is different, at least in part, because of the spirit of brotherhood and the character of the people—a statewide character at least partly forged by the hardships and challenges of the Great Depression of the late '20s and '30s, exacerbated in Oklahoma's case by the Dust Bowl. In order for people to survive, they—at least many of them—learned that they had to take care of one another, to share what they had, to understand that everyone was in it together, and if something happened to one, it could happen to all of them. The idea is that a sense of personal social consciousness is carried like a cultural memory in the minds and hearts of Oklahoma's musical artists.

If that's so, and if that spirit indeed gives Oklahoma music much of its unique character, then nowhere is the attitude better embodied than in the music that's come to be known as Red Dirt. Born in Stillwater, home of Oklahoma State University, in the 1970s, its spiritual and musical components are inseparable. Its practitioners share a strong bond that, for many, stretches back three decades or more.

Guitarist-vocalist Brad James, a longtime member of the Red Dirt jam band Medicine Show, later played in the Organic Boogie Band, which toured and recorded with Red Dirt star Stoney LaRue. He was one of many who spent time in and around a famous old house just outside the OSU campus. With acres between it and the nearest neighbors, it was a perfect place to gather and jam into the morning hours.

"All of those people who began in Stillwater gravitated around a place called the Farm, before the term 'Red Dirt' was in the newspapers and all," James explained in a 2002 interview. "It's not like the Muscle Shoals Sound or the Motown Sound. For me, it's more of a lineage thing, a community of influence."

To find the beginnings of the whole movement, however, it's necessary to go back to a time before the old two-story that would become the Farm had been taken over by a bunch of laid-back musicians always looking for an excuse to strum a guitar or pen a tune with a fellow picker. It involves a man who would, 20 years later, helm a million-plus-selling country act with roots in both Red Dirt and the Tulsa Sound.

When we had Moses back in Stillwater, it was kind of a precursor to what I'm doing today. It was that mix of Hank Williams, Chuck Berry, and Bob Dylan, that blend of country and rock 'n' roll—I don't like the term "country-rock"—that people like around Stillwater. I don't want to claim that I'm the father of the [Red Dirt] movement, but I do think we kind of coined the name for it back then.

— *Steve Ripley, 2000*

That Moses album Steve did when he was back in Stillwater was an inspiration for all of us. It empowered us. Someone did an album who was right in the neighborhood, and that made us believe that anything was possible.

— *Bob Childers, 2002*

In a 2002 conversation, Steve Ripley joked that *Moses Live*, the 1974 LP by his band at the time, "hardly made it out of Stillwater—and only in my trunk." But the disc nonetheless had a powerful effect on Stillwater's music community, as influential Red Dirt singer-songwriter Childers noted in the preceding quote. Done by Ripley's four-man group Moses and featuring an array of covers (as well as one original, Ripley's "Oklahoma Blues") taken from classic rock 'n' roll and R&B ("Shake, Rattle and Roll," "Willie and the Hand Jive"), contemporary rock and pop ("Saturday Night's Alright for Fighting," "When I'm 64") and country ("Okie from Muskogee"), it was the first release on Ripley's own label, Red Dirt Records.

Journalist Mike Dougan, in his liner notes, made what may have been the first-ever stab at defining Red Dirt music. "Red Dirt is a record company," he wrote. "It is also the color of the earth surrounding Enid [where the disc was recorded] and nearby Stillwater, Moses' home base. More important, Red Dirt is a hue of funk, a shade of sound, a basic spirit embodied in Moses' music."

Although original compositions would become an important part of the Red Dirt sound, the musical-genre mix on the Moses album not only foreshadowed the sound of Ripley's two-decades-later band, the Tractors, but also that of the Red Dirt acts that would spring up in the '80s and '90s. Although some leaned toward the honky-tonk end of things, while others let their rock influences dominate, all of the Red Dirt musicians seemed to utilize this blend of rock, country, and roots music, with a little bit of folk—especially when it comes to lyrical content—strung through it.

Ripley was a student at OSU when he played in Moses, and certainly Stillwater's status as a college town has something to do with the birth of Red Dirt. After all, college is the last bastion of irresponsibility for most kids, that time just before a person's supposed to grow up and get serious, and students usually have a lot of spare time to get into creative pursuits like music. Then, there's the fact that Oklahoma State has a longstanding reputation for its School of Agriculture, so it's always drawn a lot of students from farms, ranches, and rural areas. These are kids who were weaned on country music, and they're often thrown together in dorms and apartments with more cosmopolitan roommates who favor contemporary rock and pop. The result, for those with more than a passing interest in music, has long been a kind of cross-pollination of musical genres, out of which the Red Dirt scene emerged.

Moses was a perfect example of the influence different genres had on Stillwater musicians in the '70s, especially Ripley. But other factors in Red Dirt's birth were coming into play around the same time. John Cooper, a founding member of the Red Dirt Rangers—one of the longest-lived and most influential of the Red Dirt acts—noted in a 2000 conversation that at about the same time *Moses Live* came out, a musician named Michael McCarty "played a few times in Norman with a band called Red Dirt. It was a very short-lived experiment." McCarty, who lived in Norman, had been with the long-lived underground group the Holy Modal Rounders, best known by mainstream listeners for their song "If You Want to Be A Bird" in 1969's hit movie *Easy Rider*.

(*Oklahoma Music Guide* authors Carney and Foley cite Norman native Jesse Ed Davis, with his "Red Dirt Boogie, Brother" track on the 1972 solo album *Ululu*, as "the first Oklahoman to hint at the 'genre.'")

Moses played music that people could dance to, directly hearkening back to the days of Bob Wills and his feel-good, western-swing dance material. Soon, the music that would come to be known as Red Dirt acquired an aspect related to another Oklahoma musical ancestor, Woody Guthrie. A couple of years after *Moses Live*, the planned construction of the Black Fox nuclear power plant in Inola, about 100 miles from Stillwater, spawned a number of protests on the Oklahoma State University campus. Several musicians who'd be associated with Red Dirt music, including the man who's been called the godfather of Red Dirt, singer-songwriter Bob Childers, performed for these rallies.

"Childers even went to Washington during a [1979] rally and sang on the Capitol steps in front of 50,000 people," recalled John Cooper recently. "It was a huge national protest, and there was a big contingent from Stillwater and the Tulsa area because of Black Fox. That was a real galvanizing time for Red Dirt, because it brought a lot of people from the anti-nuke movement into the music."

So, Bob Wills' escapism and Woody Guthrie's social conscience, mixed into the musical forms of the day, became the philosophical and spiritual influences on the developing Red Dirt style. And while it could be argued that it didn't really take off until the '90s, Red Dirt was around for years before that. Bob Wiles, founding member and former bassist for the Red Dirt Rangers, relayed his point of view in a 2002 interview:

First there was Ripley and Moses, and Jimmy LaFave was coming up through Stillwater High. Before you knew it, Bob Childers and Greg Jacobs were writing great songs, and then the Skinner Brothers became the hottest band around. Then another generation comes along—like us and Medicine Show, which really champions the Red Dirt cause. Great Divide takes it to a national level. Jason Boland gets the honky-tonk revival going. Then Cross Canadian Ragweed's rockin', and Stoney LaRue's just kind of grown up on all of it, taking it all in.

Wiles' capsule history of the movement points out another important thing about Red Dirt—the idea of the music always being passed along to newer, and often younger, artists, for them to work their own ways with it.

Ripley's association with Moses, for instance, inspired singer-songwriter Jimmy LaFave, who penned the anthematic "Red Dirt Roads at Night" and has exported the Red Dirt style and attitude around the world. A member of the Austin, Texas, musical community since 1986, he nonetheless finds himself returning often to Stillwater to recharge his creative batteries.

"There's something about that part of the earth that sticks with you," he said in 2002. "I have to go back there from time to time to soak up some energy and inspiration. I plan to end up back there myself one day. I've traveled all over the planet, but my favorite place to get inspiration is traveling those red dirt roads."

Another Stillwater-based singer-songwriter, Chuck Dunlap, came along in the '70s and strongly influenced both Childers and Brad Piccolo, guitarist and vocalist for the Red Dirt Rangers. Piccolo said recently that Dunlap "was the first guy we really knew who had his own record out."

My first memory of Chuck goes back way before our band got together, back in the fall of '79, when I was driving down Highway 51 from Oklahoma

> **"IT WAS A HUGE NATIONAL PROTEST, AND THERE WAS A BIG CONTINGENT FROM STILLWATER AND THE TULSA AREA BECAUSE OF BLACK FOX. THAT WAS A REAL GALVANIZING TIME FOR RED DIRT, BECAUSE IT BROUGHT A LOT OF PEOPLE FROM THE ANTI-NUKE MOVEMENT INTO THE MUSIC."**

City to Stillwater, and I found a Stillwater station on the radio. The first song I heard was a Chuck Dunlap song, "Predestiny," and I thought, "Hey, that's a great song. I'd like to hear more of this guy's stuff."

As Bob Wiles indicated in his synopsis of the movement, following LaFave's exodus to Austin it fell to the Red Dirt Rangers and Medicine Show to carry the Red Dirt banner, something they did for several years. Medicine Show, put together by Brad James and bassist Donnie Wood in 1990, soldiered along for eight years before disbanding. At this writing, the Red Dirt Rangers were still going strong, its three remaining original members—Cooper, Piccolo and lead guitarist-vocalist Ben Han, the only Red Dirt figure to emerge from the country of Borneo—surviving a horrifying 2004 helicopter crash to continue a busy performance and recording career. At one time or another, the group's supporting members have included Tulsa Sound veterans Rocky Frisco on keyboards and Jim Karstein on drums, as well as fellow Red Dirt artists Randy Crouch on fiddle, Don Morris on bass and Kenny Early on drums. In the early part of 2006, they began recording their newest disc with Steve Ripley at Tulsa's Church Studio.

During much of the '90s, as Cooper noted in a 2000 conversation, "Childers was in Nashville and [Tom] Skinner was in Louisiana. Then, the Great Divide came along and took it more of a honky-tonk country way, which spawned Cross Canadian Ragweed and Jason Boland and the Scorchers."

Those Stillwater-based acts, once again, were inspired by the guys before them—including, and perhaps especially, the Red Dirt Rangers. The band has been such an inspiration to others, in fact, that former Rangers bassist Bob Wiles has often said, humorously, "we skipped the career and went straight to being an influence." In 2005, Cross Canadian Ragweed's Cody Canada said, "One of my goals when I moved to Stillwater [from Yukon] was to meet the [Red Dirt] Rangers, because I kind of saw 'em as the Grateful Dead of Oklahoma. They were one of those bands you look at and say, 'These guys'll be around forever.'"

"I go back with the Rangers as early as my music started," added Stoney LaRue in an interview that same year. "I've lived in Stillwater forever, and John Cooper used to play with me at Willie's twice a week. I can't remember the first time I saw them, but I do remember Brad Piccolo throwing his leg over the neck of the guitar and jumping up and down on one foot."

The Great Divide—singer and lead guitarist Mike McClure, bassist Kelley Green, and brothers Scotte (guitar) and J.J. (drums) Lester—formed in Stillwater in the early 1990s. In the late '90s, the

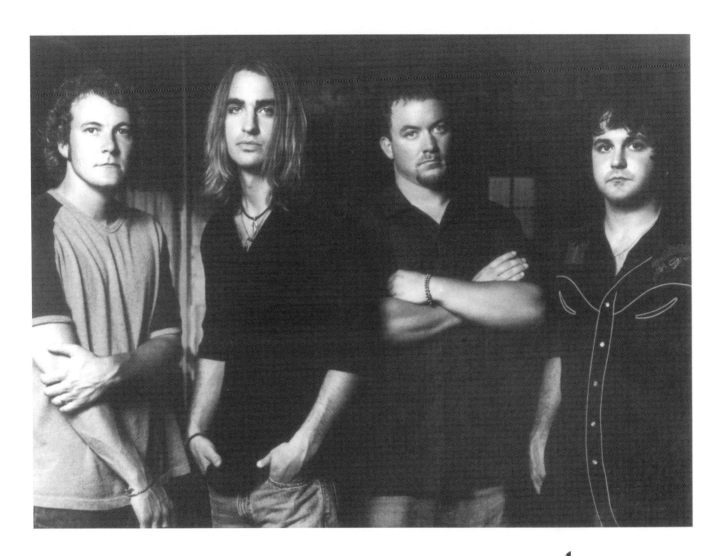

Cross Canadian Ragweed

Divide became the first of the Red Dirt acts to be picked up by a major label (Atlantic), as well as the first one to make an impact, although slight, on hit-country radio. Two of the band's songs hit the lower reaches of the national country charts in 1998, "Never Could" (rising to No. 74 on the *Billboard* Hot Country Singles chart) and the Jimmy Buffett-influenced "Pour Me A Vacation," which hit No. 59 and spawned a music video as well.

While the group left Atlantic a few years later, it continued to be a popular touring and recording act. And, as Oklahoma's second hundred years dawns, the Great Divide is still out there working, even though lead singer and primary songwriter

McClure left in 2003 to form the more rock-oriented Mike McClure Band (the outfit's first discs carry the slogan "twice as loud and half as popular"). McClure has also been producing Cross Canadian Ragweed's discs for the major label Universal South.

"I think the biggest thing we did was coming up with a style of music that was our own, and then going into clubs that demanded Top 40 covers and not doing that," McClure said in an interview just before leaving the group. "We wrote and did our own music, and when we started getting the numbers [of audience members], I think it changed things to where it wasn't the cool thing to go in and do covers anymore. I think our band was pretty instrumental in getting that done around Oklahoma."

The idea of doing original music rather than covering other people's songs is certainly an important component of Red Dirt, even though the artists often perform compositions by other writers in the movement—and by those beyond it as well. Just about any genre is fair game, too. A Cross Canadian Ragweed set, for instance, might include Ted Nugent's "Stranglehold," Bo Diddley's "Who Do You Love" and Bob Wills' "Right or Wrong." After singing Bob and Johnnie Lee Wills' "Milk Cow Blues" on a session for the 2005 disc *A Tribute to Bob's 100th Birthday*—a project put together by longtime Wills associates Leon Rausch and Owasso native Tommy Allsup—Cody Canada recalled how western swing and Red Dirt came together for him on that particular number.

I'd been singing "Milk Cow Blues" for three or four years [during his pre-Ragweed days] at the Oklahoma Opry, and then I heard the Great Divide get up and really rock it out. When we did our first album, a little demo album, we did "Milk Cow Blues" on it like the Great Divide had done it.

When Tommy [Allsup] called and asked if I wanted to do a song on the Bob Wills record, I said: "Man, that's the coolest thing anyone ever asked me." I said, "It's probably already taken, but I'd love to do 'Milk Cow Blues.'" He said: "You've got it. What key?"

Allsup, for his part, noted in a 2005 interview promoting the Wills disc that he "heard a lot of Cotton Thompson" in Canada's voice during the recording. Thompson was the vocalist on the original 1941 recording of Johnnie Lee Wills' version of "Milk Cow Blues."

After the session, Leon Raush—who became Bob Wills' vocalist in the 1950s—congratulated Canada on being the newest Texas Playboy. Canada's response: "I teared up," he said.

☙

There are those who say that despite its original sound and number of practitioners, Red Dirt is still mostly a regional phenomenon. Of course, that was true for western-swing music, too, for much of its time in the sun. Like western swing in its formative years, Red Dirt is most popular around Oklahoma and Texas, with the Red Dirt guys often given the designation of Texas Music once they cross the Red River (similar to the "western swing" and "Texas swing" appellations). To be fair, many Red Dirt acts have relocated from Oklahoma to Texas because the far-larger population of that state offers many more opportunities to play. As Stoney LaRue and others have noted, there are as many people living in the Dallas-Fort Worth area as there are in the entire state of Oklahoma.

In fact, many of the Red Dirt acts—including Jason Boland and the Stragglers, Stoney LaRue, and the fiercely independent singer-songwriter from the Tulsa suburb of Sand Springs, Brandon Jenkins—have seen their songs register significantly on the Texas Music Chart. A regional variation of the national *Billboard* magazine charts, the Texas Music Chart tracks the playlists from 80 radio stations in Texas and surrounding states, compiling and publishing the results on the website *www.texasmusicchart.com*. It's the work of a Houston-based company called Shane Media Services, which also publishes the monthly magazine *Best in Texas*.

Some have compared the Red Dirt musicians, who are often lumped with the similar-sounding Texas Music acts, to the outlaw-country artists who came along in the '70s. These singer-songwriters, including the likes of Willie Nelson, Waylon Jennings, and Jessi Colter, descended on Nashville with a new down-to-earth,

"I THINK THE BIGGEST THING WE DID WAS COMING UP WITH A STYLE OF MUSIC THAT WAS OUR OWN, AND THEN GOING INTO CLUBS THAT DEMANDED TOP 40 COVERS AND NOT DOING THAT"

uncompromising, scruffy but *real* sound that changed the whole face of country music.

So far, however, that hasn't happened—unless you count the two hit acts we'll consider in a moment as Red Dirt. Otherwise, besides the Great Divide's moderate national chart success with the two singles and an album in 1998, the only Red Dirt band that's seen some success on hit-country radio is Cross Canadian Ragweed—whose members include, in addition to lead singer and lead guitarist Canada, guitarist Grady Cross, bassist Jeremy Plato, and drummer Randy Ragsdale. Since signing with Universal South—a label co-headed by veteran record executive and native Oklahoman Tim DuBois (who's apparently still giving Oklahoma acts 25 extra points)—in 2002, CCR has had two albums hit big. *Soul Gravy*, from 2004, made No. 5 on the Billboard Top Country Albums chart (and No. 51 on the all-genre Billboard 200), while the next Universal South collection, 2005's *Garage*, hit No. 6 (No. 37 on the Billboard 200).

Despite the album successes, however, Ragweed has yet to see a major hit single, coming the closest (as of mid-2006) with the No. 39 *Billboard* country hit "Fightin' For" in '05. This relative lack of acceptance by commercial radio has little to do with the quality of Ragweed's music; instead, it's more about the group's unwillingness—despite intense pressure—to rework its sound into something that's more, as the Nashville term labels it, "radio-friendly." Because of their desire to remain true to their music in a town where musical integrity often is the first thing to drop by the wayside in the scramble for a hit, the guys in Cross Canadian Ragweed are seen as anomalies by many in the business.

The band, however, is not above having fun with that image. Tabbed to play a "Texas Music" showcase during the 2006 Country Radio Seminar in Nashville, CCR decided to go native for the occasion.

"The night before, we were talking about the show, and I said, 'You know, we ought to go out and get us some gaudy stuff and come out as Nashville sh*tkicker dudes,'" recalled Canada with a laugh in an interview shortly after that appearance. "A little later on, I come in and Randy's standing beside the bus with a big old hat and a windbreaker with 'Kenny Rogers' across the back. That's when we decided to do it.

"So we all come out [at the CRS show] in our cowboy hats and stuff. And I say, 'Well, is *this* radio-friendly enough for you?'"

I always tell people…that Austin's a great music town—which it is—and the two biggest acts to come out of here are probably Stevie Ray Vaughan and Willie [Nelson]. But then I tell 'em that between the Tractors and Garth, Stillwater's probably sold more records.

— *Jimmy LaFave*

While Cross Canadian Ragweed continues to seek country-radio success without compromising their long-held principles, a couple of Stillwater acts found themselves embraced by that same medium a decade or so earlier. We've already seen how Garth Brooks roared out of Oklahoma State University to become the biggest thing not only in country music, but all of pop music as well. And there was Steve Ripley, who began his recording career with Moses and then took a circuitous path out of Stillwater that included producing, engineering, touring and recording with Bob Dylan, and building guitars for the likes of Eddie Van Halen and Ry Cooder. He eventually returned to Oklahoma, settling in Tulsa, where he began running the venerable Church Studio—formerly the property of Tulsa Sound legend (and Ripley pal) Leon Russell, who'd had it during the halcyon Shelter Records days. In the early '90s, Ripley would join with several other Tulsa musicians to create the Tractors, a band signed by, yes, Tim DuBois to Arista Nashville.

As noted earlier, several members of this an alumnus of Bonnie Raitt's band as well as a Tulsa Sound figure who'd played with Rockin' Jimmy Byfield and other major Tulsa acts of the '70s. It was a band that combined Ripley's Red Dirt sensibilities and multiple musical influences with a group of Tulsa music vets who could play anything, and play it well.

The result was a debut disc, 1994's *The Tractors*, that sold somewhere around two million copies and spawned a bona fide hit single, the incredibly catchy "Baby Likes to Rock It," (the song David Gates, earlier in this book, cited as an example

"A LITTLE LATER ON, I COME IN AND RANDY'S STANDING BESIDE THE BUS WITH A BIG OLD HAT AND A WINDBREAKER WITH 'KENNY ROGERS' ACROSS THE BACK. THAT'S WHEN WE DECIDED TO DO IT."

group—minus Ripley and multi-instrumentalist Ron Getman—had been put together by drummer Jamie Oldaker to work behind Ronnie Dunn during the 1988 Marlboro Music Talent Roundup. Like Oldaker, whose credits included stretches with Eric Clapton, Peter Frampton and Bob Seger, the other musicians assembled for the Tractors were veterans with significant road and recording experience. Getman had played with Janis Ian and Leonard Cohen, bassist Casey Van Beek with Linda Ronstadt and the Righteous Brothers, and keyboardist Walt Richmond was of the tight shuffle "foundation of the Tulsa Sound"). With the help of an inventive video—named Music Video of the Year by the Country Music Association in 1995—the single made it all the way to No. 11 on the *Billboard* country singles chart, while the album peaked at No. 2 on the same publication's album chart, and No. 19 on the *Billboard 200*, which tracks all album sales regardless of musical genre. The Tractors also did some time on the road with Brooks & Dunn—which meant that most of Ronnie Dunn's old band found itself touring with his

Tom Skinner

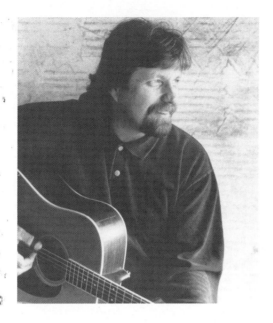

new band—and Southern country star John Michael Montgomery.

The next year, the Tractors released their second album on Arista Nashville, a seasonal offering called *Have Yourself a Tractors Christmas*. It also sold well, peaking at No. 12 on the country charts, and produced a crossover Yuletide song, "The Santa Claus Boogie."

It was three years before their third and final Arista disc would appear. *Farmers in a Changing World* came out in 1998, and despite critical acclaim, it didn't do as well as the other two albums in the country music market. It made a respectable showing, climbing into the Top 40 of *Billboard's* country chart, but its first single, "Shortenin' Bread"—supported by a music video featuring Tulsa movie actors Gailard Sartain and Gary Busey—stalled in the lower reaches of the charts.

Many of the original Tractors left around that time, but the band has continued with a number of different members and guests as a recording group, helmed by Ripley from his Church Studio. Those who've contributed to Tractors tracks over the years make an impressive array of first-rate musicians, including western-swing greats Eldon Shamblin and fiddler Curly Lewis; Elvis Presley sidemen Scotty Moore, James Burton, and D. J. Fontana; and a host of Tulsa Sound folks headed by Leon Russell. Most recently, the Tractors were associated with Audium Records in Nashville, and they were still knocking out top-flight rootsy music whose sound can at least partially, if not wholly, be classified as Red Dirt.

And then there's Garth Brooks. Some would say that he became a Red Dirt act in 1986, when he joined with several other Stillwater musicians—including bassist Tom, fiddler Mike and guitarist Craig Skinner, who'd had some collective success in the early '80s with the Skinner Brothers Band—to form the group Santa Fe.

Santa Fe, in the Red Dirt tradition, played music from both the rock and country camps, and both Brooks and Tom Skinner would become excellent songwriters as well. Prior to Santa Fe, OSU student Brooks had spent considerable time as a solo act at a Stillwater nightspot called Willie's, playing guitar and singing from a repertoire that drew from folk and rock as well as country. When the Skinners and Brooks met, as he recalled in a 2002 interview, "It was the George Strait wannabe meeting the Skinner Brothers, who did stuff like [the Lynyrd Skynyrd Southern rocker] 'I Know A Little.' So when you put those two together, like a train wreck, 'I Know A Little' becomes almost like a swing number. That's what happened.

"Stillwater somehow married all the things we loved about the '60s rock era, from Creedence [Clearwater Revival] to the Eagles to the Band, with George Strait, Asleep at the Wheel, Merle Haggard, all that *stuff*," he added. "What makes it so different and makes the Red Dirt music from Oklahoma is the addition of the Skinner Brothers to that Creedence kind of distorted sound—marrying those two things together."

The story is told earlier in this book about how Santa Fe, after a year or so of playing as a regional band, headed for Nashville and dissolved, with Brooks emerging as a solo act on his way to nearly unprecedented stardom. Although it wasn't on the same level, Tom Skinner also became a well-known singer-songwriter, ultimately moving back to Oklahoma and becoming a leading light of the Red Dirt movement. As this book is being written, Skinner is best known for his weekly Tom Skinner's Science Project events, which have been going on for several years in Tulsa. Each night's installment features Skinner and his band with a rotating cast of Red Dirt and Red Dirt-related acts, showcasing the diversity and creativity found underneath that banner.

Interestingly enough, Skinner's definition of Red Dirt music is much like Brooks'. "Really, it's all the music we grew up with," Skinner said in a 2000 conversation. "It was just sort of a natural mix. We weren't trying to invent anything." He laughed. "At least, not on purpose."

What they did invent, however, became a part of the sound of Garth Brooks, the biggest pop-music artist of the 1990s. How much of Garth's sound was Red Dirt? When asked point-blank, in that 2002 interview, if he considered himself a Red Dirt act, he answered in a typically thoughtful way.

My sound was created in Stillwater, and the sound that I took to Nashville and played—that's on every record of mine—was created in Stillwater and would not have happened without Stillwater. I'm very proud to take my place as an Oklahoma artist; I don't think I would've had this sound anywhere else. And if I hadn't run into the Skinner Brothers, I don't think you would've heard the sound we had.

Before leaving the hit-country radio stars with Red Dirt influences, we should mention again the country superstar act, Brooks & Dunn. While Kix Brooks, as noted before, is a Louisianan, and Ronnie Dunn a Texan who settled in Tulsa, the two of them wrote and recorded a tune called "Red Dirt Roads" for the 2003 disc of the same name. A nostalgic look at a rural upbringing, it deals in some of the same subject matter and attitudes that infuse Red Dirt music.

"Red Dirt Roads," incidentally, was a No. 1 country hit, as was the album.

As anyone who's written about musicians knows, they're not usually the best people to ask about how they'd classify their music. Like most artists, they don't like to be pigeonholed, and they're often too busy creating to worry about where or how what they're doing fits with what other people are doing. With that in mind, it's instructive to hear a couple of definitions of Red Dirt from folks who aren't musicians, but certainly know a lot about them.

In 2003, a young Kansan named Josh Quillan was a co-organizer of the first Red Dirt Music Awards show, which took place at Tulsa's Cain's Ballroom. Quillin had been turned onto Red Dirt music a few years earlier, when his older brother, then an OSU student, had brought home a disc by the Great Divide. Later, Quillin himself headed for Stillwater, where he found ample opportunity to soak up live performances by folks like the Divide, Cross Canadian Ragweed, and Jason Boland and the Stragglers. Eventually, he created a website, *www.reddirtscene.com*, to help spread the word.

"I may not have the most accurate definition of Red Dirt Music," he said in an interview prior, "but to me, it's not bounded by state lines."

It's guys who have taken the music from the musicians who came from this area, like Woody Guthrie, and been influenced by it—right down to people like Bob Dylan and even Willie Nelson. There isn't any set genre. It's just something they started by singing about things that were important to them, things that were on their minds, instead of singing about something some guy out there told them they needed to sing to sell records. To me, that's Red Dirt— you sing it because you love it.

As we've seen with Cross Canadian Ragweed, that attitude often puts an act at odds with the Nashville country music industry, where scoring a hit single trumps everything else. Music City resident Brandy Reed and her RPR Media have represented several Red Dirt acts, beginning with the Great Divide and continuing with Jason Boland and Cross Canadian Ragweed. In a recent interview, she said that the Red Dirt acts approach Nashville and recording in an entirely different way.

When I first started working, I had a chance to work in what they called the Music Row scene.

Then, gradually, I found myself working with Red Dirt musicians, and the difference was like night and day. The people in the Red Dirt scene have music running through their very veins. They're born to be musicians. They can't do anything else. They have an amazing respect for each other. They know each others' songs. And the best part of it is when they're on stage, jamming, heart to heart, soul to soul.

If you're around their family, their brotherhood, you get it. And when you do, it will change your life. It will change your mind about what music is supposed to be about. And at the end of the day, when the show's over and they're just hanging out and being themselves, the things they talk about and the way they love each other goes far beyond the music business.

Reed's observations reflect, among other things, the interconnectedness of the Red Dirt musicians, something the Red Dirt Rangers' Brad Piccolo sees as going back to life in Stillwater—where, he noted in 2002, "we're farther away from a big city, and we have more of a tendency to create our own fun."

As Oklahoma's centennial approaches, the Red Dirt musicians continue to create their own fun, even as their musical influence in the region and the country grows. Blending country, rock, and folk influences with intelligent, close-to-the-earth lyrics, these artists combine the Saturday night Okie abandon of Bob Wills music with the populist social conscience of Woody Guthrie. Until a better definition comes along, that may be as close as we can get to pinning down Red Dirt music. As Bob Childers, who knows as much about it as anyone, said in 2002, "I could spend the rest of my life trying to explain it. But I sure know it's there."

8
CHAPTER EIGHT
THE SECOND HUNDRED YEARS?

As Oklahoma's centennial year approaches, acts from the state are once again making big noises in country music. Clinton native Toby Keith—who, as we've seen, started charting national hits in the early '90s—finally hit the top rung of the ladder just about the time the new millennium began. In 2000, he was the Academy of Country Music's Male Vocalist of the Year, and in 2001 he took home the same honor from the Country Music Association. Then, in 2003, he became the ACM's Entertainer of the Year. At least partially on the strength of his two-fisted flag-waver, "Courtesy of the Red, White and Blue (The Angry American)," the album *Unleashed* debuted at No. 1 on the *Billboard 200* chart in 2002, ultimately going multiplatinum. According to Carney and Foley in *Oklahoma Music Guide, Unleashed* was only the eighth country album to reach the top of that all-genre *Billboard* chart—and the other seven were from fellow Okie Garth Brooks.

Brooks, for his part, remained committed to his retirement from an active country music career, although he authorized the giant Wal-Mart chain to repackage his first six albums, adding previously recorded but unreleased material, into a boxed set called *Garth Brooks: The Limited Series*. Later, a single-CD collection called *The Lost Sessions* was spun off from the set, with six previously unreleased tracks added. Although sales of both titles couldn't be tracked through regular channels, they undoubtedly added a few million to his already stratospheric totals, as well as providing significant mailbox-money income to some of the writers of those previously unreleased cuts. Red Dirt singer-songwriter Mike McClure, for instance, finally cashed some nice checks for his composition "I'd Rather Have Nothing," cut by Garth years before but unreleased before the new collections. As of mid-2006, other releases of previously recorded Brooks material were expected from Wal-Mart.

Brooks also recorded a couple of new songs, both of which could be seen as coming under special circumstances. In late 2005, he cut a tribute to his late pal and fellow musician Chris LeDoux, "Good Ride Cowboy," which became a Top Five hit. Then, in 2006, he and new wife Trisha Yearwood recorded the duet "Love Will Always Win," which made it into the country-music Top 25.

Yearwood, a Georgia native, had been a country hitmaker since 1991's "She's in Love with the Boy." By the time 2005's *Jasper County*—her first album in five years—came out, she'd settled in the Tulsa area with Brooks. The disc soared to No. 1 on Billboard's Top Country Albums chart, eventually going gold (signifying sales of 500,000 copies) and yielding the country radio hit "Georgia Rain" and the Top 30 adult-contemporary single, "Trying to Love You." Her career rejuvenated, Yearwood has joined the ranks of Oklahoma-based country stars.

"The nice thing about living here is that it's incredibly normal," she said in a 2005 interview. "It's really nice to go back to Nashville and get my job done and then come back here."

Picher's Joe Don Rooney, a vocalist, guitarist, and songwriter, got his start with the now-defunct Grand Lake Opry, located in the northeastern Oklahoma resort town of Grove. A decade or so later, he's one-third (with Ohio cousins Jay DeMarcus and Gary LeVox) of the hit-country superstar group Rascal Flatts, known for monster singles like "These Days," "What Hurts the Most" and "I Melt" (whose video became famous for showing a flash of Rooney's bare backside). After winning the CMA's Horizon Award—given for career growth—in 2002, the band became the CMA's Vocal Group of the Year in '03, '04 and '05, with the ACM also recognizing Rascal Flatts as Top Vocal Group in 2005.

In the early part of the decade, the trio—augmented by other musicians—had been a reliable opening act that had once toured with Toby Keith, among others. However, by 2005 the band was a solid headliner, with a highly successful road show featuring a couple of Oklahoma recording artists, Ada's Blake Shelton ("The Baby," "Some Beach") and Miami's Keith Anderson ("Pickin' Wildflowers," "Every Time I Hear Your Name") in support. In August of '05, the three acts played just outside of Anderson's hometown at the Buffalo Run Casino, an event that drew more than 17,000 and snarled traffic for miles.

"Joe Don and I were talking about it," said Anderson in an interview later that year. "There were more people at that concert than there are in both our towns combined. It was a big concert in a soybean field behind the casino. You don't get much more Oklahoma than that."

You don't get much more Oklahoma than Checotah's Carrie Underwood, either. The charismatic young woman put her hometown—and her college, Northeastern Oklahoma State University in Tahlequah—on the national radar in 2005, thanks to her all-the-marbles triumph on the hit television show *American Idol*. Her weekly

> **"THERE WERE MORE PEOPLE AT THAT CONCERT THAN THERE ARE IN BOTH OUR TOWNS COMBINED. IT WAS A BIG CONCERT IN A SOYBEAN FIELD BEHIND THE CASINO. YOU DON'T GET MUCH MORE OKLAHOMA THAN THAT."**

exposure as an *American Idol* contestant and eventual winner translated nicely to her recording career. Even before her first album was released, she'd set a record by being the first country artist to have a song debut at No. 1 on the *Billboard Hot 100*, the all-genre singles version of the *Billboard 200* album chart. That distinction belonged to "Inside Your Heaven," a song she'd done on the TV show that was rushed into release.

Several weeks later, Underwood's *Some Hearts* hit No. 1 on the Billboard country albums chart, the fastest-selling debut disc ever from a new country artist. That torrid sales pace continued for months afterward, and in early 2006 Underwood also became the country artist to go triple-platinum (signifying sales of three million) in the shortest amount of time.

Some Hearts' first single, "Jesus, Take the Wheel," spent several weeks at No. 1, with the next song from the album, "Don't Forget to Remember Me," achieving hit status as well. Although it may never be a single, "I Ain't in Checotah Anymore" should be mentioned here. The only track Underwood co-wrote on *Some Hearts*, it contains the lines "I'd rather be tippin' cows in Tulsa than hailing cabs here in New York." The way things are going with her high-flying career, however, she may be doing a lot more of the former than the latter over the next stretch of years.

Carrie Underwood

We've already looked at Red Dirt, an Oklahoma-spawned musical movement that's still very much on the upswing. Its impact on the national music scene can't yet be calculated and its history is yet to be written, but if an act like Cross Canadian Ragweed or Jason Boland and the Stragglers were to become a force on the country-music charts, and the artists considered earlier in this chapter continued to cut hit records, Oklahoma performers could once again crowd under the country-music spotlight in a force and profusion not seen since the early '90s golden age of Garth, Vince, Reba, and Ronnie.

What other musical movements will wend their ways out of Oklahoma and across the world during Oklahoma's second hundred years? Will a new kind of rock music, like the Tulsa Sound in the '70s, spring from the state? One could argue that it may have already happened with the Flaming Lips, a band that came out of the Norman-Oklahoma City area post-punk rock scene in the early '80s to, as the *Tulsa World's* Mark Brown recently wrote, "defy odds, buck tradition and, with a rare combo of work ethic and strange genius, stand mysteriously apart."

Jim DeRogatis, the *Chicago Sun-Times* pop critic who recently wrote a book called *Staring at Sound* about the improbably long-lived band, told Brown that the band's Wayne Coyne is "a genius."

"He's the cowboy who has the really great thoughts and expresses them in an educated way," said DeRogatis. "He's Will Rogers."

Even though the Flaming Lips have been major-label artists since 1992, they still seem to be on the rise. The past couple of years have seen not only the emergence of the DeRogatis book and a well-received documentary about the band called *The Fearless Freaks*, but also a new Warner Bros. disc, *At War With the Mystics*, that just missed the Top Ten of the *Billboard 200*.

As is the case with Cross Canadian Ragweed and the other Red Dirt artists, it's too early to tell if the Flaming Lips will end up having a major influence on their musical contemporaries, or be at the vanguard of any particular sound. The same is true for Tulsa's Wayman Tisdale, the pro basketball star turned jazz artist. Playing lead bass with his Fifth Quarter Band, Tisdale has not only cut seven CDs for various labels—including 2001's *Face to Face*, a No. 1 disc on *Billboard's* Contemporary Jazz Albums chart—but helped along other smooth-jazz acts in and around his hometown, including Tulsa-based saxophonist Eldredge Jackson, whose album Tisdale produced, appeared on, and co-wrote. If Tisdale turns out to be in the forefront of an Oklahoma-based contemporary-jazz sound, it would be an intriguing reflection of the music that put the state on the musical map back in the 1920s and '30s.

Of course, there are many other talented performers now, some just beginning their careers in front of audiences, others woodshedding in Oklahoma garages and living rooms, struggling to develop a sound that's all their own. Some of those sounds may someday influence the world, perhaps even catalyze their own musical movements. And as the Dust Bowl and Great Depression recede and finally disappear from anyone's living memory, one can only pray that their lessons stick. Just as Oklahoma's music continues, growing and changing, gathering influences from all over and taking them in unique and creative directions, so should the brotherhood and character and social conscience and empathy continue right along with it, as the state moves into a second hundred years of life, hope, and music.

ADDENDA

HALLS OF FAME AND HALL OF FAMERS

Because this book has been concerned with the musical trends and genres that began in Oklahoma and grew to have an impact on popular music far beyond the state's borders, Oklahoma performers who aren't a part of any greater movement have generally remained outside of its parameters. That fact, it should be emphasized, doesn't mean to slight in any way the significant individual achievements of pop-music greats like Patti Page and Kay Starr, noted songwriters like Jimmy Webb and Kevin Welch, Broadway performers like Kristin Chenoweth and Sam Harris, opera stars like the acclaimed Leona Mitchell, or even Nokie Edwards and Bob Bogle, founders of the Ventures, the most successful instrumental rock group of all time. It also doesn't mean to downplay the contributions of many Oklahoma rock and pop artists to the contemporary-Christian music scene over the past few decades, stretching back to the beginnings of trumpeter Phil Driscoll's career in the genre, and up to the likes of Christian hard-rock group Pillar.

What all this *does* mean, simply, is that those artists, and scores of others, are subjects for different books, ones concerned more with individuals than movements. Carney and Foley's *Oklahoma Music Guide*, cited numerous times in this text, is one of those books, as is William W. Savage's *Singing Cowboys and All That Jazz: A Short History of Popular Music in Oklahoma* (University of Oklahoma Press, 1983).

Beyond those volumes, and this one, further information on the depth and breadth of Oklahoma acts can be gleaned by taking a look at the inductees into the state's music-oriented halls of fame. The Oklahoma Jazz Hall of Fame, located in Tulsa, has been inducting music figures since 1989, while Muskogee's Oklahoma Music Hall of Fame came up with its debut class in 1997. Then, in 1999, the *Tulsa World* newspaper, in conjunction with its Friday entertainment magazine, *Spot*, threw the first of its annual awards shows, recognizing top local and state performers and including at least one Hall of Fame induction per year.

Here, then, are the inductees into each Oklahoma music hall of fame, with a line or two of biography accompanying any artist who hasn't been adequately identified before in these pages.

Chuck Cissel is himself a worthy hall of fame candidate. A singer and dancer on Broadway—he was a member of the Tony-winning cast of *A Chorus Line*—Cissel also recorded as a solo act for the MCA and Arista labels (with his 1980 album *Just for You* going Top 40 on Billboard's Black Albums chart), and led his own West Coast combo for several years. In 2000, he returned to his hometown of Tulsa, where he became CEO of the Oklahoma Jazz Hall of Fame, even as he continued to perform.

"The first thing is that most of the jazz hall inductees are from the state of Oklahoma, born and raised here—or, if they weren't, they must've lived here for more than 25 years," said Cissel recently.

We go out and look for these cats—on the East Coast, the West Coast, the Midwest. Some of our inductees look out for us and send in names of people they know. It's like, "You may not know this guy, but here are his credits, and he's from Oklahoma." And we go, "Wow."

That's how we find people like [inductees] Louie and Maurice Spears. They're from Oklahoma City, and while many people may not know them, they're nationally known in music circles and very well respected.

There aren't a lot of set criteria for a potential inductee into the jazz hall, although the musician has to have made his or her mark in jazz, blues, or gospel music, with an appearance on at least one album or CD. Otherwise, it's up to the Oklahoma Jazz Hall of Fame board members on the illumination committee.

"Names are tossed into the hat, and we discuss what they've done, what they've achieved, and if they've been good ambassadors for the state of Oklahoma, and not just on a self-absorbed musical trip," Cissel explained.

Non-Oklahoman artists are represented in the hall via honorary inductions, or as recipients—along with a few of the state's major stars—of either the Living Legend Award or the Jay McShann Lifetime Achievement Award. "Most of the Living Legends and Jay McShann Lifetime Achievers aren't from here," noted Cissel. "Those honors are our attempt to expand the roster to include those [non-Oklahomans] we respect for their musical accomplishments, people like Dave Brubeck, Louie Bellson, and Jon Hendricks. They come in and do shows and master classes for us, and it gives us a more national exposure."

He smiled. "I saw a poster for Ramsey Lewis' 'Legends of Jazz' show, and it listed him as a Grammy Award winner and recipient of the Oklahoma Jazz Hall of Fame's Lifetime Achievement Award."

Here, then, are the musical honorees in the Oklahoma Jazz Hall of Fame through 2005, listed chronologically, with brief explanations for those not already mentioned. Since 2002, a Legacy Tribute Award has also been given to an artist from the state who, in Cissel's words, "has created an outstanding level of musical work for a given year that warrants special accolades." These honorees are listed as well.

INDUCTEES TO THE OKLAHOMA JAZZ HALL OF FAME

1989

ZELIA PAGE BREAUX *The longtime music supervisor for Oklahoma City's black schools, her students included Jimmy Rushing and the Christian brothers, Edward and Charlie.*

CHARLIE CHRISTIAN

ERNIE FIELDS *A Tulsa-based trombonist and bandleader, Fields' best-known work was done on the West Coast in the late '50s and early '60s, when the Ernie Fields Orchestra had a No. 4 Billboard pop hit with a reworking of Glenn Miller's "In the Mood."*

LOWELL FULSON *This Tulsa-born bluesman wrote the classic "Everyday I Have the Blues," put a number of singles in the Top 10 of the rhythm & blues charts, and toured with his own band, which, in the early '50s, included pianist Ray Charles.*

JAY McSHANN

JESSIE MAE RENFRO SAP *A gospel-music performer for decades, Oklahoma City native Sapp made a big impact in the gospel market as a Peacock Records artist in the '50s. Her album* He's So Wonderful *spent more than three years on the* Billboard *gospel chart.*

CLAUDE WILLIAMS

1990

THE BLUE DEVILS

AL DENNIE *A busy musician with territory bands like the Bennie Moten and Paul Banks outfits, this Wellston native organized the Jap Allen Band and led his own group as well.*

CLARENCE LOVE

JIMMY RUSHING

C. C. SKINNER *A gospel songwriter and nationally known choir director, Tennessee native Skinner was minister of music for Tulsa's Paradise Baptist Church for 30 years and, in the '70s, founder of the North Tulsa Singing Convention.*

1991

CHET BAKER *Trumpet and flugelhorn player and vocalist, Yale-born Baker became, in the '50s and '60s, the king of the West Coast cool-jazz scene.*

JOEY HOBART CRUTCHER *a minister of music and director of such Tulsa-based choirs as the Love Connection and Unlimited Praise, Crutcher is also the longtime music director of the Northeastern Oklahoma chapter of the Gospel Music Workshop of America.*

BARNEY KESSEL

CECIL McBEE *Bassist McBee, a Tulsa native, played in New York with such top jazzmen as Wayne Shorter and Yusef Lateef in the '60s, and then began leading his own jazz band, later founding the group The Leaders and continuing to play with a number of big-name artists.*

ROY MILTON *Born in Wynnewood, vocalist-drummer Milton grew up in Tulsa, where he appeared on radio station KVOO,* played with Ernie Fields' aggregation for a few years, and then moved to California, where he formed the Solid Senders, a pioneering jump-blues outfit. Later, he recorded several R&B hits as a solo artist for the famed Specialty label.

1992

SAMUEL AARON BELL

KENNETH E. KILGOR Leader of the Ambassadors' Concert Choir, an Oklahoma City-based group from St. John Missionary Baptist Church. Under Kilgore's direction, it became a nationally known interfaith choir.

JOE LIGGINS Guthrie native Liggins was a pianist, vocalist, and bandleader who scored a million-selling hit with 1945's "The Honeydripper," an instrumental recorded by his group the Honeydrippers. Liggins also recorded other '40s rhythm & blues hits and had a long run as both a touring and recording act.

HONORARY (NON-OKLAHOMAN) INDUCTEES:

RUTH BROWN AND DUKE ELLINGTON

1993

EARL BOSTIC Saxophonist and arranger Bostic, a Tulsa native, made his recording debut with Lionel Hampton in 1939 and spent a year with Hampton's orchestra before going out on his own, successfully mixing jazz and R&B and recording and performing extensively with his own combos.

ELMER L. DAVIS Director of sacred music for Tulsa's Paradise Baptist Church, Davis also spent 10 years as the vocal music director for Tulsa Public Schools.

JIMMY LIGGINS Younger brother of 1992 inductee Joe, this Newby-born guitarist and singer also recorded for the Specialty label, cutting several R&B hits with a group called the Drops of Joy. According to the Oklahoma Music Guide, the Drops of Joy's 1948 single "Cadillac Boogie" is considered by some to be the first-ever rock 'n' roll record.

LEE SHAW Shaw is a jazz pianist from Cushing whose nationally released albums include 1996's Essence and 2002's Place for Jazz.

HONORARY INDUCTEE:

DIZZY GILLESPIE

1994

HOBART MELVIN BANKS Born in Rentiesville, Banks was a pianist who worked with a number of regional and territory bands, including groups led by Muskogee's Leonard Howard, Oklahoma City's Bucky Coleman, and Tulsa's Ernie Fields. His resume included a one-week engagement at Harlem's famed Cotton Club.

VERBIE GENE "FLASH" TERRY Guitarist-vocalist Terry, an Inola native, toured with a number of nationally known blues and R&B acts in the '50s and '60s, but he's best remembered as one of Tulsa's leading blues players for nearly a half-century, driving a city bus by day and playing music by night. A beloved figure in his hometown, Terry was also instrumental in the development of the Tulsa Sound, as he welcomed young white rock 'n' rollers to north Tulsa clubs like the Flamingo, where they could experience first-hand the blues and R&B that influenced their own music. "If you were a musician or a music fan, you could come in there and sit down," he recalled in a 2003 conversation. "I'm tellin' you, I didn't know segregation back then—in the Flamingo Club, for sure."

FLOYD RICHARD WILEY A child prodigy in his Tulsa hometown, Wiley was a gospel-music arranger, composer and keyboardist who worked with several groups out of the Friendship Missionary Baptist Church and taught music in the Tulsa and Beggs school systems for more than two decades.

HONORARY INDUCTEE:
THOMAS A. DORSEY
LIVING LEGEND AWARD:
DOROTHY DUNEGAN

1995

OSCAR PETTIFORD Recognized as one of the greatest jazz bassists who ever lived, Okmulgee native Pettiford began working with national names like Charlie Barnet, Roy Eldridge, and Coleman Hawkins in the early 1940s, spending significant time with big-band stars Duke Ellington and Woody Herman before becoming known for his appearances with jazzmen like Stan Getz and Thelonious Monk in the '50s.

JOHNNY ROGERS Rogers is probably best known for his jump-blues work with fellow Oklahoman Roy Milton in the '40s, when Rogers was the guitarist for Milton's Solid Senders.

MARSHALL ROYAL Born in Sapulpa, saxophonist Royal is known best for his two decades as a featured member of Count Basie's group, beginning in the early '50s. Recently, an annual jazz festival bearing his name began in the town of his birth.

HONORARY INDUCTEE:
MAHALIA JACKSON
LIVING LEGEND AWARD:
MILT HINTON

1996

ERNIE FIELDS JR. Son of the Tulsa-based bandleader inducted into the first Oklahoma Jazz Hall of Fame class, the younger Fields is a noted West Coast session musician and producer.

BILLY HUNT This Grove-born trumpeter played with big-band icons Harry James (three years) and Woody Herman (12 years), winning a Grammy for his "Days of Wine and Roses" solo with Herman's outfit.

MELVIN MOORE Another former Ernie Fields sideman, Oklahoma City native Moore was a trumpeter and vocalist who went on to play with Jimmie Lunceford in the '30s and

'40s and Dizzy Gillespie and Charles Mingus in the '50s and '60s, among many others.

JIMMY NOLEN *Oklahoma City's Nolen was the longtime guitarist in the J.B.'s, James Brown's famed backing band, during the latter part of the '60s and most of the '70s.*

HAROLD SINGER *Another former member of Ernie Fields' Tulsa-based band, Singer went on to a career as an R&B vocalist, with his '50s hit "Cornbread" giving him a nickname that stuck.*

WALTER "FOOTS" THOMAS

--- **1997** ---

DON BYAS

OSCAR ESTELL *Vocalist and saxophonist Estell, born in Tulsa, worked with the territory bands of Clarence Love and Ernie Fields, and later with the likes of Lionel Hampton, Sam Cooke, and Art Farmer.*

TONY MATHEWS *A Checotah native, guitarist-vocalist Mathews has spent time with the bands of Ray Charles and Little Richard and carved out a recording and touring career for himself as a solo artist. He often headlines at the annual Dusk Till Dawn Blues Festival in Rentiesville, an event begun by fellow bluesman and 1999 Oklahoma Jazz Hall of Famer D.C. Minner.*

MATTHEW MCCLARTY *A gospel music figure from Ada, McClarty was the first African American to perform on his hometown radio station. Much later, in 1982, he and his group appeared as a part of the Smithsonian Folklife Festival in Washington, D.C.*

HONORARY INDUCTEE:

ELLA FITZGERALD

--- **1998** ---

ELVIN BISHOP *Although he's a contemporary of many of the first-generation Tulsa Sound artists, guitarist-vocalist Bishop didn't really begin playing until he left town to go to college in Chicago, where he quickly immersed himself into that city's blues scene. Bishop's achievements include co-founding the influential Paul Butterfield Blues Band in the early '60s, a million-selling pop hit ("Fooled Around and Fell in Love") in 1976, and a number of albums for a variety of labels.*

CLARENCE DIXON *Born in Texas, Dixon came to Tulsa as a child and lived most of his life there, working with Ernie Fields' band from 1931 through 1947. Despite the fact that the Fields group was a territory band, only occasionally venturing out of the Southwest and Midwest, Dixon came in second in the jazz-drummer category in a 1940* Downbeat *magazine poll.*

ERNESTINE DILLARD *A powerful Tulsa-based soprano, known for her soaring vocals, gospel artist Dillard has sung for audiences across the country and performing for some United States presidents.*

WASHINGTON RUCKER *A Tulsa native, Rucker is a drummer whose extensive* *credits range from bebop pioneer Dizzy Gillespie to pop and R&B superstar Stevie Wonder. Among other things, he played on the acclaimed Ray Charles and Cleo Laine recording of Gershwin's* Porgy and Bess.

LIVING LEGENDS AWARDS

GEORGE FAISON (non-performing category)

and

LOUIE BELLSON

1999

KEN DOWNING *A legendary Tulsa bandleader and saxophonist, his influence on the town's jazz scene from the late '50s through the '70s was immense. Just about every jazz player in town spent time with Downing's big band at one time or another, including fellow inductees Steve Wilkerson, Andrea Baker, and Pat Kelley, all of whom were college students when they joined Downing's outfit.*

D.C. MINNER *A veteran blues guitarist and vocalist who toured with the likes of Chuck Berry, Jimmy Reed and fellow inductee Lowell Fulson, Minner is best known in Oklahoma for converting his Rentiesville birthplace to the Down Home Blues Club. He and his bassist wife, Selby, run the club and, in the same location, the annual Dusk Till Dawn Blues Festival. They've also been very active in Oklahoma Arts Council programs in the public schools, teaching kids about the blues.*

PAT MOORE *Inducted in the gospel category, Tulsa-based pianist and vocalist Moore is also a proficient jazz player. At age 9, she was playing for the Paradise Baptist Church's senior choir, and began working professionally in area clubs in the late '60s.*

DAVID T. WALKER *Tulsa native Walker was a West Coast session guitarist who worked with top acts ranging from Marvin Gaye to Pharoah Sanders and recorded several LPs under his own name. Of those, 1976's* On Love *was the most successful, climbing onto the jazz, pop and R&B charts.*

MAXINE WELDON *This blues-jazz vocalist and Tulsa native cut her first albums in the early 1970s, seeing R&B chart action with 1974's* Some Singin'. *Her more recent efforts include starring in the successful touring show* Wild Women Revue.

LIVING LEGENDS AWARD

LINDA HOPKINS

LIFETIME ACHIEVEMENT AWARD

JAY MCSHANN (a native Oklahoman)

2000

HELEN BAYLOR *Born in Tulsa, vocalist Baylor was raised in Los Angeles, where she opened for such acts as Aretha Franklin and Stevie Wonder. She recorded her first gospel album in 1990, at the age of 35, quickly becoming a fixture on the contemporary-Christian and gospel music charts.*

KAY STARR *A major '50s pop-music recording artist, Dougherty's Starr broke into the big time with Joe Venuti's orchestra while still in her mid-*

teens. She also worked with famed big-band names Glenn Miller, Charlie Barnet and Bob Crosby before beginning a solo career that yielded such huge pop hits as 1952's "Wheel of Fortune" and 1955's "Rock And Roll Waltz," among many others.

TED TAYLOR *Vocalist Taylor, born in Okmulgee, made his biggest national impression in the mid-'60s to mid-'70s, when he recorded a number of R&B singles including 1966's "Stay Away from My Baby," which rose to No. 14 on the* Billboard *Black Singles chart.*

LEE WILEY *Fort Gibson native Wiley was a highly respected jazz singer, making her first big impact as a radio vocalist in New York during the '30s. She was also a lyricist and recording artist who cut whole albums devoted to the work of a single composer—something unusual in those days—beginning in 1939 and 1940 with 78 rpm collections of George Gershwin and Cole Porter compositions.*

JAY MCSHANN LIFETIME ACHIEVEMENT AWARD:

JON HENDRICKS

2001

WAYNE BENNETT *Bennett, who grew up in Oklahoma, recorded with the likes of Jimmy Reed, Buddy Guy, and Magic Slim. He then became a part of Chicago's Blues Consolidated Revue, along with Bobby "Blue" Bland. It was the beginning of a decades-long association between vocalist Bland and guitarist Bennett.*

GLENN E. BURLEIGH *A Guthrie native, Burleigh was the director of music for the National Baptist Congress for five years, as well as composer-in-residence for the Ambassador's Concert Choir in Oklahoma City. His composition "Order My Steps" was a nominee for Song of the Year in the 1995 Dove Awards.*

THE BURTONS *The husband and wife team of Charles and Barbara Burton have been playing music together for more than three decades. Tulsa natives, vocalist Barbara and guitarist-vocalist Charles live and work in Oklahoma City. Individually, their credits include the Jazz Messengers (Barbara) and Gladys Knight and Tom Jones (Charles).*

SONNY GRAY *A Tulsa jazz institution, Gray is known not only for his piano playing, but also for owning the legendary Rubiot, the '60s Tulsa jazz club, where both local and national jazz luminaries would come to sit in with his combo.*

JOHN HENRY *Although he appeared regularly with the rock 'n' roll revival act the Bop Cats, Tulsa rock historian and longtime deejay Henry was a blues inductee in the non-performance category. The induction came from his long-running* Smokehouse Blues *radio show, which debuted in 1987 on Tulsa's KMOD—with syndication to other area stations—and featured both live and recorded music.*

JAY MCSHANN LIFETIME ACHIEVEMENT AWARD:

LOU DONALDSON

2002

WILLIE EARL CLARK *Saxophonist and vocalist Earl Clark and his band, Spectrum, have been a fixture on Tulsa's entertainment scene for many years. In addition to performing extensively in the area, he also works as a music instructor for Tulsa Public Schools and with the Oklahoma Jazz Hall of Fame.*

JESSE ED DAVIS

CARLTON PEARSON *Minister and major-label recording artist, Pearson led his Tulsa-based Higher Dimensions Choir through three albums on the Warner Alliance and Atlantic Records label. He was also the presiding Bishop of more than 600 churches and ministries affiliated with the Azusa Interdenominational Fellowship of Christian Churches and Ministries, Inc,*

LIVING LEGEND AWARD:

PATTI PAGE *(a native Oklahoman)*

JAY MCSHANN LIFETIME ACHIEVEMENT AWARD:

DAVE BRUBECK

LEGACY TRIBUTE AWARD:

WAYMAN TISDALE

2003

PAT KELLEY *Tulsa's Kelley settled on the West Coast, where he became a top-notch session guitarist, playing on records, tours, and in the television orchestras of such stars as Merv Griffin and Carol Burnette. His credits range from work with B.B. King to Donny and Marie Osmond, and his own discs include 1989's* I'll Stand Up, *which was a Top 25 entry on Billboard's* Contemporary Jazz Albums *chart.*

SARA JORDAN POWELL *Inducted in the gospel music category, vocalist Powell has performed all over the world, and is especially known for her performance before Mother Teresa.*

LESLIE SHEFFIEL *A contemporary of and frequent collaborator with members of the Oklahoma City Blue Devils, this Muskogee-born pianist, composer and arranger worked in the Oklahoma City-based Rhythmaires Band, which featured a young Charlie Christian. According to Sheffield's jazz hall biography, Christian brought one of Sheffield's compositions, "Flying Home," with him to the Benny Goodman Orchestra. Goodman is officially credited with composing the famous tune.*

LIVING LEGEND AWARD:

TAJ MAHAL

JAY MCSHANN LIFETIME ACHIEVEMENT AWARD:

MARILYN MAYE

LEGACY TRIBUTE AWARD:

JACOB FRED JAZZ ODYSSEY *(Nationally known, Tulsa-based contemporary jazz group)*

2004

TOMMY CROOK *Often performing solo or with only a bassist, Crook is Tulsa's best-known* nightclub guitarist. Eschewing the touring life, he nonetheless received a measure of national fame when Chet Atkins praised him on *The Tonight Show* in the '70s.

Jimmy "Cry Cry" Hawkins
A major area blues act in the '50s, vocalist Hawkins was not only a staple of the club scene on Tulsa's Greenwood Avenue, but also gave many local players their start.

Frank Mantooth
Pianist and college-level educator Tulsa's Mantooth is perhaps best known for his innovative jazz compositions and arrangements, many of which are used in music programs across the country.

Louie and Maurice Spears
Bassist and cellist Louie and bass trombonist Maurice, brothers hailing from Oklahoma City, put their classical training to use as first-call West Coast musicians and music educators, playing on movie and TV soundtracks and working with stars ranging from Neil Diamond to Horace Silver.

Glenn R. Townsend
A blues and blues-rock figure on the Tulsa club scene for many years, guitarist-vocalist Townsend is best known for the big Texas blues-style sound created by his three-piece band.

LIVING LEGEND AWARD:

Stanley Jordan

JAY MCSHANN LIFETIME ACHIEVEMENT AWARD:

Ramsey Lewis

LEGACY TRIBUTE AWARD:

Grady Nichols
(Tulsa-based smooth-jazz saxophonist)

2005

Andrea Baker
A Muskogee native, vocalist Baker has appeared with such jazz and big-band greats as Stan Kenton, Billy May and Jack Shelton, and toured and performed with many other musicians, including her saxophonist husband and fellow inductee, Steve Wilkerson. She also has extensive credits as a voice teacher and music director, and has produced albums for several artists.

Madeline Manning Mims
Inducted in the gospel category, Tulsa' Mims first came to national attention as an Olympic gold medalist, setting a record in the 800-meter run. From there, she became a concert, television, and recording artist with an international ministry.

David Skinner
A Tulsa resident since 1980, Texas native Skinner was a part of the early '70s Austin scene, playing with the likes of Stevie Ray and Jimmie Vaughan, Lou Ann Barton and Johnny Winter. A singer and guitarist, he played in a number of bands, including his own, after settling in Tulsa.

Steve Wilkerson
Wilkerson's first job came at the age of 11 in the town of Ramona, when he joined his father's dance band. Since then, he's become famous for his work on tenor sax, recording on his own and with others,

including his vocalist wife Andrea Baker. Like Baker, he's also a sought-after music educator.

LIVING LEGEND AWARD:
FREDDY COLE

JAY MCSHANN LIFETIME ACHIEVEMENT AWARD:
NAT "KING" COLE

LEGACY TRIBUTE AWARD:
ELDREDGE JACKSON

The Oklahoma Music Hall of Fame, located in a historic former Frisco train depot in Muskogee, inducted its first group of musicians in 1997, following the creation of a group called Friends of Oklahoma Music and a resolution by the Oklahoma State Legislature designating Muskogee as the site of the hall. Each year since, the Muskogee Civic Center has hosted an annual Oklahoma Music Hall of Fame Induction Ceremony and Concert, in which many of that year's honorees perform, often with an added headline act. A group of electors that includes board members, current hall of famers, music-industry personnel, music scholars, and media figures is responsible for nominating each year's potential honorees.

The eligibility requirements are listed under "Induction Criteria" on the group's website, *www.oklahomamusichalloffame.com*:

Along with having made significant and noticeable contributions to the field of music, to be considered for induction into the Oklahoma Music Hall of Fame, a nominee should have some solid connection to the state of Oklahoma, either by birthright, moving to the state at an early age, living in Oklahoma for a significant portion of his or her career, writing songs or music about Oklahoma, or furthering music in the state of Oklahoma. Excellence in the field of music will be the primary criteria for induction into the Oklahoma Music Hall of Fame.

Also included in its induction standards is a statement that the hall, "(g)iven the unique history of American Indian music in Oklahoma," will induct the 38 American Indian "tribes, bands, and nations of Oklahoma who have persisted in their musical traditions," with the order of induction based on each group's date of arrival at what is now Oklahoma. These inductions are made every fourth year, and they're included in the following list. The group also occasionally gives other special awards, including the Rising Star Award and the Governor's Award.

INDUCTEES TO THE
OKLAHOMA MUSIC HALL OF FAME

1997

WOODY GUTHRIE

MERLE HAGGARD *The country-music icon known as "the Poet of the Common Man" was a natural for the hall for several reasons, not the least of which was his 1969 monster hit, "Okie From Muskogee." His parents worked a farm in Checotah until Dust Bowl-era circumstances forced them out of the state and on the road to California. It's generally acknowledged that Haggard was born in a boxcar in Bakersfield, but a rumor persists that he's actually a Checotah native, born before his parents made the trek West.*

PATTI PAGE *A Claremore native, Page was one of the first and most successful country-pop crossover artists, with her 1950 chart-topper "Tennessee Waltz" still the biggest-selling single by a female artist of all time. Over the next couple of decades, she charted dozens of other hits on both the pop and country charts, including such well-remembered numbers as "Doggie in the Window," "Allegheny Moon," and "Old Cape Cod." One of the first vocalists to overdub her own voice on her records, Page was also a trailblazing television star.*

CLAUDE "FIDDLER" WILLIAMS

1998

GENE AUTRY

ALBERT E. BRUMLEY *Born near Spiro, Brumley was a leading gospel music figure who wrote more than 600 gospel songs and hymns, including such standards as "I'll Fly Away," "Jesus, Hold My Hand," and "Turn Your Radio On."*

DAVID GATES

JAY MCSHANN

1999

BYRON BERLINE *Born in Kansas but raised in Oklahoma, champion fiddler Berline played in such well-known bluegrass groups as the Dillards and Bill Monroe & the Bluegrass Boys before heading to the West Coast, where he—among other things—helped create the California country-rock sound with groups like Sundance, Dillard & Clark and the Flying Burrito Brothers. At this writing, he lives in Guthrie, where he hosts the annual International Bluegrass Festival.*

VINCE GILL

BARNEY KESSEL

KVOO—*The former home of Bob Wills was the first radio station inducted into the hall.*

2000

THE BLUE DEVILS

ROY CLARK

COLOR ME BADD *Bryan Abrams, Mark Calderon, Sam Watters and K.T. Thornton met as students at Northwest Classen High School in Oklahoma City, and went on to international fame in the early '90s with such pop-chart hits as "I Adore Mi Amor," "All 4 Love" and* the notorious "I Wanna Sex You Up," which appeared on the soundtrack of the film New Jack City and went on to sell millions of copies.

JIM HALSEY

WANDA JACKSON

2001

CADDO INDIAN TRIBE

LEONA MITCHELL Enid native Mitchell is a superstar soprano who has sung dozens of roles on opera stages all over the world. According to the Oklahoma Music Hall of Fame, she "achieved international recognition when she was selected to sing Bess in the London Records complete recording of the George Gershwin classic Porgy and Bess with the Cleveland Orchestra."

BOB, JOHNNIE LEE, LUKE, and BILLY JACK WILLS, and THE TEXAS PLAYBOYS

2002

CHARLIE CHRISTIAN

JOE DIFFIE

KAY STARR

HANK THOMPSON

2003

RONNIE DUNN

BENNY GARCIA, JR.—Oklahoma City native Garcia was a jazz guitarist capable of playing with Benny Goodman—which he did—but his best-remembered work came with major western-swing figures like Tex Williams and Hank Penny before World War II, and Bob and Johnnie Lee Wills afterward.

FLASH TERRY

D.C. MINNER

LEE WILEY

JOHN WOOLEY

2004

DR. LOUIS BALLARD Composer and pianist Ballard, born near Quapaw, has seen his work performed all over the world, with premieres at such prestigious venues as Carnegie Hall and Lincoln Center. Primarily known for his compositions in the classical style, including the ballet The Four Moons, Ballard was also producer, director, and composer for the first all-Indian halftime show, presented at Washington, D.C.'s Robert F. Kennedy Stadium.

MERLE KILGORE Chickasha native Kilgore wrote or co-wrote such country-music classics as "Wolverton Mountain," "More and More," and "Ring of Fire." He also managed Hank Williams Jr. for a long stretch and was an officer in both the Country Music Association and the Nashville Songwriters' Association International.

ROGER MILLER Born in Texas, Miller grew up in a farm near Erick, where he was befriended by Sheb Wooley, who'd go on to a good career as a singer, songwriter and actor himself. Miller's big break came in 1958, when Ray Price recorded his "Invitation to the

Blues," but Miller is best known for his string of novelty crossover hits in the '60s—"Dang Me," "King of the Road," "Kansas City Star" and many more—and, later, for scoring the Broadway musical "Big River," for which he won two Tony Awards.

2005

TOMMY ALLSUP *Cain's Ballroom—Like the powerful AM station KVOO, inducted in 1999, the Cain's Ballroom provided a home for decades for the bands of Bob and Johnnie Lee Wills. Unlike KVOO-AM, the Cain's Ballroom still exists as a viable musical force.*

TOBY KEITH

BILLY PARKER *Influential as both a much-honored disc jockey and a recording artist, Tuskegee's Parker has been the voice of country music in Oklahoma for more than 30 years, many of them spent on KVOO-AM. Recipient of Disc Jockey of the Year Awards from both the Country Music Association and the Academy of Country Music, Parker continues to make new friends and fans with his broadcasts, recordings, and live shows.*

In 1999, the first Spot Music Awards were held in Tulsa at the Cain's Ballroom, a venue especially fitting since Bob Wills became the first member of the Spot Music Hall of Fame on that night. The awards, given in a number of different categories annually ever since, are named after *Spot*, the Friday entertainment magazine of the *Tulsa World*.

"Anybody can vote on the awards," said Cathy Logan, editor of the Tulsa World's Scene section, recently. "The votes come mostly from our readership area, but we've had ballots that came from as far away as Australia and Great Britain."

The Hall of Fame selections, she added, are picked in a different way. "It's the consensus of the entertainment staff at the *Tulsa World*," she explained. "We argue it out, but we generally come to an agreement. We take lasting influence into consideration. We look at people who didn't just have a hit record, but helped to shape the music that came behind them. We want to recognize those people whose work was really influential in shaping the music of others, who had an influence on the rich stew of the state's music."

Sometimes, she said, even those who cover Oklahoma music aren't fully aware of the connections between past and present musicians. She cited an instance at the 2000 event, when a young Tulsa rapper and his group stood and cheered wildly when the late Johnnie Lee Wills received the second Spot Music Hall of Fame designation.

"That night," she recalled, "he told me, 'Of course we know the music of Johnnie Lee Wills. That's where we came from.'"

Artists who have won five times in a particular category are also automatically inducted into the

Spot Music Hall of Fame. Those who became hall of famers via that route are noted in the following list of inductees, complete through 2005.

SPOT MUSIC HALL OF FAME

-1999
Bob Wills

-2000
Johnnie Lee Wills

-2001
Leon Russell

-2002
Patti Page
Barney Kessel

-2003
Flash Terry
Steve Ripley

-2004
Roy Clark
Red Dirt Rangers
   (five-time winners in Best Red Dirt Act category)

-2005
Steve Pryor
   (veteran Tulsa guitarist and vocalist with major-label experience who was a five-time winner in Best Blues Act category)

Jacob Fred Jazz Odyssey
   (five-time winner in Best Jazz Act category)

ALSO BY JOHN WOOLEY

FICTION

Ghost Band

Awash in the Blood

Dark Within

Death's Door (with Ron Wolfe)

Full Moon (with Ron Wolfe, as by Mick Winters)

Old Fears (with Ron Wolfe)

Thrilling Detective Heroes (editor, with John Locke)

Roscoes in the Night (editor, with John Gunnison)

At the Stroke of Midnight (editor)

Robert Leslie Bellem's Dan Turner, Hollywood Detective (editor)

NON-FICTION

Voices from the Hill: The Story of Oklahoma Military Academy

The Big Book of Biker Flicks (with Michael H. Price)

How To Make it in the Music Business (with Jim Halsey)

Forgotten Horrors 4: Dreams that Money Can Buy (with Michael H. Price)

Forgotten Horrors 3: Dr. Turner's House of Horrors (with Michael H. Price)

Hot Schlock Horror

Forever Lounge (with Thomas Conner and Mark Brown)

SCREEN

Cafe Purgatory

Dan Turner, Hollywood Detective (The Raven Red Kiss-Off)

Hauntings Across America

Still Swingin'

Sourdough, Beefsteak & Beans

COMICS & GRAPHIC NOVELS

The Twilight Avenger

The Miracle Squad

The Uncanny Man-Frog

Plan Nine From Outer Space

Plan Nine From Outer Space: Thirty Years Later

Tor Johnson, Hollywood Star

Dan Turner, Hollywood Detective